HYPOTHERMIA, FROSTBITE and other COLD INJURIES:

HYPOTHERMIA, FROSTBITE and other COLD INJURIES:

Prevention, Recognition, and Prehospital Treatment

James A. Wilkerson, M.D., Editor
Merced, California

Cameron C. Bangs, M.D.
Oregon City, Oregon

John S. Hayward, Ph.D.
Victoria, British Columbia

with the assistance of
Mark J. Tuttle
Merced, California

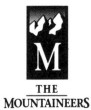

THE
MOUNTAINEERS

The Mountaineers: Organized 1906 "... to explore, study, preserve, and enjoy the natural beauty of the northwest."

Published by The Mountaineers
1011 S.W. Klickitat Way, Suite 107
Seattle, WA 98134

Published simultaneously in Canada by
Douglas & McIntyre, Ltd.
1615 Venables Street, Vancouver, B.C. V5L 2H1

Manufactured in the United States of America

Library of Congress Cataloguing in Publication Data
Wilkerson, James A.
    Hypothermia, frostbite, and other cold injuries.

    Includes bibliographies and index.
    1. Hypothermia.   2. Frostbite.   3. First aid in
illness and injury.   I. Bangs, Cameron C.   II. Hayward,
John S.   III. Title. [DNLM: 1. Cold--adverse effects.
2. Frostbite.   3. Hypothermia. WD 670 H998]
RC88.5.W49 1986   616.9'88'1   86-690
ISBN 0-89886-024-5

8 7 6 5 4

7 6 5 4

Contents

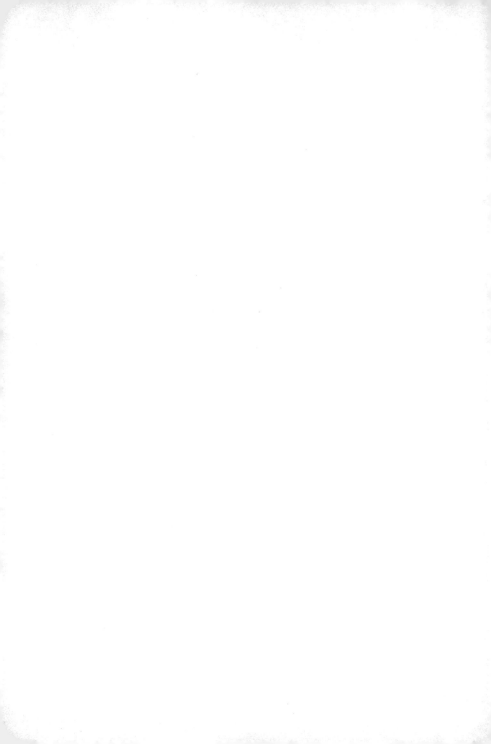

Acknowledgments

John Pollock, who was Director of The Mountaineers Books at the time, originated the idea for this monograph, because he thought a replacement was needed for the Mazamas' pamphlet *Hypothermia: Killer of the Unprepared* after the death of its author, Dr. Ted Lathrop. Without his urging and the continued support of Donna De-Shazo, who followed him at The Mountaineers Books, this book would have never been completed. Ann Cleeland and Steve Whitney, who share the position of Editorial Manager for The Mountaineers Books, also provided encouragement and assistance. Steve carried out the final editing of the manuscript with skill and insight.

The contributors, Cam Bangs, an internist in Oregon City, Oregon, who is widely known for his expertise in the diagnosis and treatment of cold injuries, and John Hayward, Professor of Biology at the University of Victoria, Victoria, British Columbia, who has carried out numerous experimental studies of immersion hypothermia, have generously allowed their portions of the text to be edited into a uniform style more appropriate for the audience to which this material is directed. They have also assisted in other ways—advising about the general content of the book, providing much information for chapters other than the ones they have written, and supplying the illustrations. Mark Tuttle, who founded and directs Tuttleworks, a wilderness clothing and equipment manufacturer, has been an invaluable source of information about equipment and garments for cold weather use and the materials from which they are made.

Finally, I would like to acknowledge the love and support of my family and their acceptance of the time directed to this undertaking, without which this little book could not have been written.

James A. Wilkerson, M.D.

The authors and publisher offer in good faith the information regarding the prevention and treatment of hypothermia and cold injuries as described in this book. This information is not intended as a substitute for specific training and practical experience to develop the skills and judgment needed for administering treatment wisely. Readers also should be aware that the information provided in this book is intended for use in the contexts described. The authors and publisher disclaim any liability for injuries that may result from the use, correct or otherwise, of this information.

The Mountaineers

Introduction

JAMES A. WILKERSON, M.D.

The Four Inns walk, an annual competitive hike over the English moors, is forty-five miles (73 kg) long, with a total ascent of about 4,500 feet (1,400 m). In 1964 this competition was held in weather that appropriately can be described as disastrous. A heavy rain was falling. Wind speeds as high as twenty-nine miles per hour (47 kph) were measured at sea level, and even stronger winds were probably encountered on the moors. Temperatures ranged from freezing to slightly above (32° to 45° F or 0° to 7° C).

Two hundred and forty hikers attempted the course. Only twenty-two finished. (Usually two-thirds of the competitors finish.) Three hikers died of hypothermia. Four others were rescued in critical condition.

This tragedy attracted much attention. Many contemporary outdoorsmen are surprised to learn how little was known about hypothermia at the time of this competition, which took place just over twenty years ago. Even the term "hypothermia" was unfamiliar, and deaths caused by cold weather or immersion in cold water were attributed to "exposure" or "freezing." Fortunately, the deaths of these hikers created an awareness of the danger of hypothermia and led to a realization of the need for more knowledge about this problem. As a result a number of studies were carried out, many of them by Griffith Pugh, a physiologist who had been a member of the 1953 British Mount Everest expedition.

One of the more obvious lessons from the analyses of this event was the inadequacy of the clothing worn by the participants. The clothing of the hypothermia victims provided less than forty percent of the insulation they were later calculated to need. The clothing worn by most of the other participants was equally inadequate.

Another lesson was the inadequacy of the food consumed by the hikers for maintaining a high level of physical activity. The total energy expenditure by the hikers who finished the course was calculated to be 6,000 kilocalories, but most of the participants had a caloric intake estimated to be only about 1,000 to 1,500 kilocalories.

However, the most surprising discovery was the inability of most participants to generate enough heat by physical exercise to match their losses to the severely cold environment. Even though all of the hikers had been selected because they were in top physical condition, most could not maintain an exercise level that would produce the heat required to keep them warm. Without clothing that significantly reduced heat loss, only the strongest hikers could keep up a pace which protected them from the cold. (The winners finished in average times.)

Cold weather recreational activities ranging from high altitude mountaineering to ice fishing continue to increase in popularity. Associated with these avocations is a constant risk of cold injuries, predominantly hypothermia and frostbite. Although hypothermia has become a familiar term, many outdoorsmen, justifiably proud of their strength and endurance, still think they can power their way through severely cold conditions such as those encountered on the 1964 Four Inns walk.

Preventing cold injuries is entirely preferable to treating them; improper treatment seems inexcusable in light of the widely available information about these disorders. This monograph has been written to provide an understanding of the effects of cold on the human body so that outdoorsmen can avoid cold injuries. Unfortunately, some individuals do not seem to appreciate the need for such precautions. Furthermore, accidental cold injuries can occur in spite of adequate preparations. (Who can foresee falling into a creek?) Therefore, a discussion of the recognition and prehospital treatment of cold injuries is also included.

Because this material is directed to an audience with a variable background, Fahrenheit temperatures have been used with equivalent centigrade (Celsius) temperatures listed in parentheses, usually rounded to the nearest full degree. More exact Fahrenheit to centigrade conversions have not been provided because the decimal fractions are cumbersome and the temperatures at which physiologic events occur are not so precisely defined.

An effort has been made to avoid medical terminology or "jargon." However, a few terms are so basic for an understanding of cold injuries that they could not be entirely eliminated. Definitions for these terms are provided below. Because an understanding of these terms is so essential, this brief glossary has been placed at the front of the book instead of in an appendix, as is customary.

GLOSSARY

Core—The central or "core" tissues of the body, generally considered to consist of the vital organs, particularly the heart, lungs, liver, and brain.

Distal—More remote or at a greater distance from the center of the body (from Latin *distans,* to be remote).

Frostbite—A localized cold injury characterized by freezing of the tissues.

Hypothermia—A lower than normal temperature (from Greek *hypo,* less than, under, or reduced, and *therme,* heat).

Hypothermic—Having a lower than normal temperature.

Hypoxia—A condition in which oxygen concentrations are lower than normally found at sea level.

Hypoxic—Having a lower than normal oxygen content; usually used to describe blood or air.

Normothermia—A normal temperature (from Latin *norma,* rule).

Normothermic—Having a normal temperature.

Periphery—The peripheral tissues of the body, generally considered to consist of the skin and subcutaneous fat of the trunk and all of the tissues of the arms and legs.

Proximal—Nearer the central part of the body (from Latin *proximus,* nearest).

Vasoconstriction—Blood vessel constriction (from Latin *vas,* a vessel).

Vasodilatation—Dilatation of blood vessels.

ADDITIONAL READING

Pugh LGCE: Deaths from exposure on Four Inns walking competition, March 14-15, 1964. *Lancet* 1964;1:1210-2.

CHAPTER ONE

Human Body Temperature and Its Control

JAMES A. WILKERSON, M.D.

Man is a warm blooded mammal. Because his body temperature is relatively constant he is called "homothermic," or "homeothermic" (Greek *homos*, the same; Greek *homoios*, like or similar; Greek *therme*, heat). He is also called "endothermic" (Greek *endo*, within) because most of the heat which maintains that constant temperature comes from the metabolism of nutrients within his body, an important consideration in avoiding cold injuries. In contrast, cold blooded, or "poikilothermic," animals have a body temperature which varies considerably and are considered "exothermic" because much of their body heat is derived from their environment (Greek *poikilos*, many colored; Greek *exo*, without).

The normal human body temperature is usually said to be 98.6° F (37° C), but this value is actually an average of oral temperatures in healthy persons. Normal temperature can be as low as 96.5° F (35.8° C) or as high as 100° F (37.8° C). Furthermore, a person's temperature usually varies 1.25° to 3.75° F (0.7° to 2.1° C) during each twenty-four hour period. The body temperature of an individual who is active during the day and sleeps at night is usually lowest in the early morning, 3:00 to 5:00 A.M., and highest in the late afternoon or early evening. The average variation is 2.7° F (1.5° C) for men and 2.2° F (1.2° C) for women. Additionally, women's body temperatures vary with their menstrual cycles, suddenly rising about 1.0° F (0.5° C) at the time of ovulation and staying at that level until menstruation begins. (Relying upon that rise in body temperature to indicate the occurrence of ovulation, and abstaining from sex at that

1

time, is a form of birth control—the rhythm method—that is about eighty percent effective.) During prolonged vigorous exercise, such as competitive distance running, a normal, healthy person's temperature can increase dramatically because he is producing heat faster than it can be lost. Temperatures as high as 104° F (40° C) are not uncommon, and in hot, humid conditions, which impair heat dissipation by sweating, higher temperatures and heat illnesses, such as heat stroke, occur.

TEMPERATURE CONTROL

Humans are able to maintain an almost constant body temperature in spite of wide swings in the temperature of their environment. This control is achieved in two ways: through "physiologic" responses that increase or decrease heat loss and can not be voluntarily controlled, and by deliberate, intellectually derived, voluntary actions to obtain greater protection from heat or cold than physiologic responses alone can provide.

When the body is resting, almost all of the energy from food metabolism ultimately appears as heat. About 1,000 calories (one kilocalorie) per kilogram of body weight per hour are produced. Since the body is composed mostly of water and has a specific heat similar to water, the body temperature would rise about 1.8° F (1.0° C) per hour if no heat were being lost. Man evolved in the tropics and had to develop adaptations to a climate which could be hot but was rarely cold. His physiologic mechanisms for increasing heat loss are more highly developed than mechanisms for conserving heat or increasing its production, and heat constantly is being lost in all but uncomfortably hot, humid environments.

At environmental temperatures between 82° and 93° F (28° and 34° C), the ambient air is warm enough to pose no threat of chilling a nude adult human body and is cool enough to absorb the heat the body produces without requiring metabolic work, such as sweating, to aid in its loss. This range of temperatures has been labeled the thermoneutral zone. At higher environmental temperatures sweating must be initiated because heat production can not be reduced below the quantity generated by vital functions.

At lower environmental temperatures maintaining a normal body temperature usually requires that heat loss be reduced. Increasing heat production with muscular activity can help maintain a normal temperature but the amount of heat that can be generated, even by vigorous muscular activity, is small in comparison to the amount that can be lost in a severely cold environment. Unrelieved immersion in cold water or exposure to low temperatures and high winds without adequate protective clothing usually results in lethal hypothermia in spite of strenuous exercise by well conditioned individuals.

Involuntary Changes in Heat Loss

Heat which must be lost is generated within the body by muscles performing physical work and by metabolic chemical reactions taking place predominantly in the liver. Most of this heat (approximately ninety to ninety-five percent) is dissipated through the skin, although smaller amounts are lost through the lungs. (The lungs are a major pathway for heat loss in panting animals such as dogs.) Although some heat is conducted directly, most of the heat produced by the muscles and liver is transferred by warming the blood which circulates through them. This blood subsequently is circulated through the skin where its heat is transferred to the atmosphere (or to water if the body is immersed). The cutaneous blood vessels, by contracting or dilating to control the flow of blood through the skin, determine how much heat is lost. The blood flow through maximally dilated cutaneous blood vessels is 100 times greater than the flow through vessels tightly constricted to minimize heat loss. At such high flow rates the temperature difference between the deep tissues and the skin is virtually abolished, and heat loss is greatly increased.

The amount of heat transported by the circulatory system is augmented by increases in the blood volume. When humans enter a hot environment, fluid moves from the tissues into the blood, increasing its volume by as much as ten percent.

Heat loss is also greatly increased by sweating, particularly in a dry climate. Changing one gram of water (as perspiration) on the skin from a liquid to a gas extracts about 580 calories from the underlying tissues. That heat loss would lower the temperature of 580 cc of water 1° C, or would lower the temperature of one liter of water 1° F. Clearly, large amounts of heat can be lost this way. In fact, heat dissipation through sweating is essential for survival at environmental temperatures above 95° F (35° C). Heat illnesses such as heat stroke result largely from inadequate heat loss. In a very humid environment sweat does not evaporate, leaving the individual "dripping with perspiration" and reducing heat loss to dangerously low levels. A severely dehydrated person may be so depleted of fluids that water for sweating is not available, again leading to greatly diminished heat loss.

(The different ways heat is removed from the skin surface are considered in Chapter Two, "Avoiding Hypothermia.")

Heat loss is reduced by mechanisms opposite to those that increase heat loss. The most significant is constriction of the blood vessels. Narrowing of vessels in the skin closes off the flow of blood through the "radiator." Not only is heat loss from the skin reduced, but the skin (with the underlying tissues) becomes a cool outer shell that reduces heat loss from the deeper tissues. Additionally, all of the blood vessels to the extremities contract. Since those structures are thinner cylinders with a relatively larger surface area, heat loss from them is greater than from the trunk. Reducing the blood flow helps diminish such heat loss.

Involuntary Changes in Heat Production (Shivering)

The only effective way adult humans can increase heat production is by increasing muscular activity. Metabolic heat production in other tissues may be increased briefly by the hormones adrenaline and noradrenaline (epinephrine and norepinephrine), but the quantity of heat produced is insignificant in comparison with the quantities required to warm the entire body. To significantly increase heat production the body resorts to shivering, a familiar response which consists of uncontrolled, irregular, and incoordinated contractions of the voluntary muscles.

The mechanisms that control shivering are incompletely under-stood but include sensors in the skin and in the brain. A drop in the core temperature initiates vigorous shivering. Cooling of the skin without a significant change in core temperature can also initiate shivering. Furthermore, warming the skin of a hypothermic indi-vidual can make him stop shivering even though his core temperature has not changed. Finally, a hypothermic individual usually stops shivering when his core temperature falls below 90° to 92° F (30° to 31° C). These responses are considered in more detail below.

Heat production during shivering can be as much as five times greater than heat production at rest. Therefore, shivering tends to slow the drop in body temperature in a hypothermic situation and serves as a warning of the need for measures to prevent hypothermia. However, not all of the effects of shivering are beneficial. An indi-vidual would be better off performing useful work, such as hiking out of the threatening situation, if he knew where he was and where he needed to go. Furthermore, much more heat can be produced by voluntarily exercising the larger muscles, such as those in the legs. Finally, shivering interferes with coordinated movements and can deplete the muscles of nutrients such as glucose or glycogen that would be needed for voluntary activities.

Shivering is decreased by alcohol, tranquilizers, low blood sugar, or high altitude. Ingestion of these drugs, exercising to exhaustion, or altitude hypoxia predispose an individual to hypothermia by in-hibiting shivering as well as by impairing intellectual function.

Body Size and Heat Loss

Because most heat is lost through the skin, the ratio of the area of the skin surface to the volume of the body determines the speed with which heat is lost. Small bodies have a significantly larger surface to volume ratio than large bodies.

The differences in these ratios can be illustrated with cubes measuring one inch and two inches on each side. The one inch cube has a volume of one cubic inch (1 in X 1 in X 1 in or [1 in]³), a surface of six square inches (1 in X 1 in X 6), and a surface to volume ratio of 6:1 or six. The larger two inch cube has a volume of eight cubic inches (2 in X 2 in X 2 in or [2 in]³), and a surface of twenty-four square inches (2 in X 2 in X 6), but a surface to volume ratio of 24:8, or only three.

As a result of the proportionally greater surface area of their skin, babies, children, and even small adults can lose heat considerably faster than larger individuals in identical situations. For the same reason, heat is lost faster from the extremities than from the trunk.

Regulation of Temperature

The involuntary mechanisms that determine heat loss and heat production are regulated—turned on and off and finely balanced—in two ways. The dominant control is exerted by temperature control centers ("thermostats") located in an area at the base of the brain known as the hypothalamus. However, blood vessels in the skin are capable of reacting to temperature changes even when the nerves connecting them with the brain have been cut, so cutaneous control mechanisms must also exist.

The posterior portion of the hypothalamic thermoregulatory center controls heat retention by decreasing heat loss and increasing heat production. If this portion of the center is destroyed, an animal can not conserve heat when it is in a cold environment but loses heat normally when it is warmed. The anterior portion of the center has opposite functions and is known as the "heat loss center." If this portion of the brain is destroyed, an animal can maintain its temperature in a cold environment but can not lose heat in a hot environment. Damage to this center in humans by a stroke or a tumor produces the rare disorder known as "malignant hyperthermia," in which the body temperature soars to lethal levels unless it is controlled with water baths or similar measures.

The thermal regulatory centers function much like a thermostat and respond to information they receive from two sources: the temperature of the blood which bathes the brain, and impulses from nerves originating in the skin. Generally, the information from these two sources is integrated to generate the most beneficial response, although an input from only one can initiate a change. For example, an immobile person immersed in cold water begins to shiver as his skin temperature falls, even though his core temperature—and therefore the temperature of the blood circulating through the brain—is still normal. If he remains in the cold water, his core temperature soon falls in spite of the shivering. If he is subsequently removed from the cold water and placed in a warm bath, he stops shivering as soon as his skin becomes warm, even though his core temperature may still be falling.

Voluntary Changes in Heat Loss

Humans have rather severe functional limitations when compared with many other animals. Most individuals do not have the physical strength of mammals their size, nor do they have the speed or endurance. They do not have the visual acuity, the discriminatory sense of smell, or the sensitive hearing of many animals. More relevantly, they can not tolerate cold water immersion like seals or other aquatic mammals.

However, humans do have unique intellectual abilities with which they can compensate for their physiologic limitations. Man uses his intelligence to protect himself from cold by engaging in voluntary physical activity, designing and wearing protective clothing, constructing shelters, and manipulating sources of heat such as fire. Describing such behavior is a major objective of this publication. Clothing for cold environments is discussed in Chapter Two, "Avoiding Hypothermia." Behavior that diminishes the hypothermia resulting from cold water immersion is considered in Chapter Seven, "Immersion Hypothermia."

Humans are not the only animals who have developed behavior that provides protection from cold. Migration to warmer climates and hibernation are two well known behaviors used by other species.

Adaptation to Cold

Certain peoples have an incredible tolerance for cold. Charles Darwin described women of Tierra del Fuego nursing their babies in open boats with no apparent discomfort, while snow fell on their bare breasts. The aboriginals of central Australia are renowned for their cold tolerance. They can remain asleep after their core temperature has begun to fall, which allows them to sleep on the cold ground. Nonaboriginals almost inevitably wake up when their core temperature drops. In spite of a number of investigations, cold adaptation in these and similar groups is not understood.

Adaptation to a cold environment by animals is found only in species that have evolved in such environments. Man evolved in the tropics and moved to cold climates only as he developed the intelligence to move a tropical microclimate of clothing, shelter, and fire with him. Adaptation to cold that would provide significant protection from hypothermia would not be expected and has not been observed in individuals who have grown up in temperate climates.

Resting body metabolism rates and the secretion of thyroid hormones are mildly increased in inhabitants of cold climates, but not enough to be protective.

All newborn placental mammals, including human infants, have deposits of fat tissue known as "brown fat." Within the cells of this tissue, fat is stored as multiple small droplets instead of one large globule, as in ordinary fat cells. Brown fat cells also contain numerous large mitochondria, the energy producing structures of all cells. Unlike ordinary fat cells which can only store fat, these cells are capable of metabolizing fat in response to hormones such as insulin and epinephrine or in response to sympathetic neural stimulation. In laboratory animals—mostly rats—these cells have been found to play a critical role in producing heat in a cold environment and in avoiding obesity, because they can metabolize fat at a very rapid rate without having to perform some other associated function, as do muscle cells, for instance. Large quantities of brown fat are retained into adulthood in all small placental mammals, particularly hibernators. However, in humans brown fat largely disappears shortly after birth and can not be regenerated in response to cold exposure. Although brown fat plays a major role in temperature regulation in newborn humans, its role at later stages of life remains uncertain.

One type of adaptation to cold that has been observed in humans is "cold vasodilatation," or the "hunting reaction." When the hands are immersed in water cold enough to damage the skin, the blood vessels constrict to preserve heat. However, at periodic intervals (about every seven to fifteen minutes) the blood vessels dilate, particularly in the fingers, allowing a much greater blood flow, which warms the tissues. This vasodilatation, which can be seen and felt because the skin of the hands becomes pink and feels warmer, serves to protect the fingers from cold injury and disability. Cold vasodilatation is increased by acclimatization to cold and partially explains why cold water fishermen, Lapps, Eskimos, and similar people can work with bare hands for long periods of time in conditions most others find intolerable.

Cold vasodilatation does have some adverse consequences, however. Heat loss is increased, particularly if the entire body is immersed in cold water.

MEASURING BODY TEMPERATURE

Temperature is measured with thermometers, most of which contain a material which either expands or sends out a greater electrical current as it is warmed. Mercury, a metal that is liquid at environmental temperatures, expands in a relatively uniform manner when it is heated. Mercury thermometers are inexpensive, easy to carry, and accurate. However, they require several minutes to register the actual temperature, and are made of glass and easily broken. Clinical thermometers are mercury thermometers with a valve that inhibits the return of mercury to the bulb and reduces the delay before the actual temperature is indicated. Prior to use, such thermometers must be "shaken down" to return enough mercury to the bulb for the indicated temperature to be below that being measured.

Electronic thermometers as they are warmed increase either the voltage emitted by paired metals or the electrical resistance. Such thermometers are accurate, easier to read, and register temperature much faster than mercury thermometers. A discardable sheath over the probe eliminates the problem of sterilization between patients. Electronic thermometers are too expensive and too bulky to be routinely carried into wilderness areas but probably should be carried by rescue groups anticipating hypothermia victims. Within recent years a variety of tapes which change color or otherwise indicate temperature have been developed. These are useful for screening for an elevated temperature, but no such devices that measure temperatures in the hypothermic range are currently available.

Most clinical thermometers are designed to measure an increase in body temperature—a fever or hyperthermia—and only go down to about 94° F (34.4° C). For situations in which subnormal body temperatures are anticipated, thermometers which can measure temperatures as low as 75° to 80° F (24° to 27° C) are desirable. Several sources for such thermometers are listed in the Appendix.

If a low reading thermometer is not available, an ordinary atmospheric thermometer can be used with certain precautions. It must be read while it is in the patient's mouth or immediately after removal because the indicated temperature begins to drop at once. Taking the temperature of a person who is not hypothermic can give an indication of the thermometer's accuracy.

Body temperature can be measured most readily by placing an oral thermometer beneath the tongue. (The average body temperatures cited are based on oral measurements.) Mercury thermometers must be left for about three minutes. Measuring oral temperatures with glass thermometers is unsafe if the patient is not fully conscious and cooperative. If the thermometer is bitten and broken, the glass fragments can produce severe injuries.

Rectal temperatures are usually about 1.0° F (0.5° C) higher than oral temperatures and more accurately reflect body core temperature. The thermometer should be lubricated and inserted two to three inches into the rectum. Due to their inconvenience, particularly outdoors in bad weather, rectal temperature measurements are rarely obtained outside of a hospital or similar situation. However, they can be a valuable aid in evaluating the hypothermic patient. Some other way of measuring the temperature must be found if the patient is thrashing about. Injuries resulting from a broken glass rectal thermometer could be life threatening in a remote wilderness situation.

Axillary (armpit) temperatures are about 1° F (0.5° C) lower than oral temperatures, but can be used when temperature measurements can not be obtained from other sites because the patient is injured or uncooperative. An oral or rectal thermometer should be placed in the armpit and the arm held against the side of the body for two to three minutes. Axillary temperatures are less reliable because they are so variable. They are not precise enough for early detection of temperature changes in patients with febrile illnesses, but they are accurate enough for evaluating hypothermic patients in a wilderness setting. Core temperature is roughly 2° F (1° C) higher than the axillary temperature. An axillary temperature of 93° F (34° C) indicates only mild hypothermia.

Tympanic membrane (ear drum) temperature measurements reflect body core temperature accurately, but require special equipment and are used only for investigative studies.

Most groups encountering hypothermia in the wilderness are not equipped with thermometers, which commonly break or malfunction in any case. Decisions concerning the patient's condition and treatment must be based on the signs and symptoms he presents, not solely on a measured temperature. In order to be prepared for handling such problems, outdoorsmen must be familiar with the typical features of both mild and profound hypothermia.

CHAPTER TWO

Avoiding Hypothermia

JAMES A. WILKERSON, M.D.

Man must act consciously and intelligently to protect himself from hypothermia in any environment which has a temperature below that of the thermoneutral zone. Two actions are possible: reducing heat loss and increasing heat production.

HEAT LOSS

Heat is lost from the skin in four ways: convection, conduction, evaporation, and radiation. In the temperate surroundings in which most people live and work, fifty to sixty-five percent of the heat of metabolism is lost by radiation. Most of the remainder is lost through evaporation. Most clothing made of currently available materials does not effectively reduce these forms of heat loss.

In contrast, convection is often the major source of heat loss in a cold environment, particularly if the air is moving. Heat loss by convection can be enormous in a strong wind. Conduction is a major route of heat loss during cold water immersion. Fortunately, heat loss by convection and conduction can be effectively reduced with currently available clothing materials.

Convection

Convective heat loss occurs whenever air—or water—that has a temperature below that of the body comes into contact with the skin and subsequently moves away. While in contact with the body, the air is warmed. Cool air that replaces it also must be warmed. The heat which warms the air is lost whenever the air moves away.

Convection is the way soup is cooled by blowing on it. The air just above its surface is warmed by the soup. Blowing moves this warm air away and replaces it with cool air which extracts more heat as it is warmed. Fans have been used since ancient times to take advantage of the cooling effect of moving air.

The amount of heat lost by convection is determined by the temperature difference between the air and the body surface with which it is in contact and by the speed with which the air is moving. The greater the temperature difference the larger is the heat loss. However, little heat is required to increase the temperature of air (its specific heat is low), and low temperatures are well tolerated in still air.

Of far greater significance to individuals who are outdoors is the ability of air in motion to remove large quantities of heat. In a wind the amount of heat lost increases as the square of the velocity—not in proportion to the velocity. A wind of eight miles per hour (12.8 kph) removes four times as much heat—not twice as much—as a wind of four miles per hour (6.4 kph). (At wind speeds above thirty miles per hour [48 kph] heat loss does not increase very much because the air does not stay in contact with the body long enough to be warmed to skin temperature.)

"Wind chill" is a term coined for the additional cooling produced by wind in a cold environment. The accompanying wind chill chart was derived from work published in 1945 by Paul Siple, who carried out many physiologic studies during Admiral Byrd's Antarctic expeditions. Siple compared the time it took water to freeze at different temperatures and wind conditions. Those conditions with similar freezing times were considered equivalent. The resulting values are not precisely correct for human bodies, which are composed of more than water, but time has proven this chart to be an accurate indicator of the additional cooling produced by wind. It also demonstrates the manner in which temperatures which pose little threat to healthy, warmly clothed persons in calm air, such as 15° F (-9° C), can be life threatening in a wind of twenty to twenty-five miles per hour (32 to 40 kph).

Table 1. Wind Chill Chart

Wind   *Temperature (Fahrenheit/Centigrade)*

(Miles per hour)
(Kilometers per hour)

CALM	35	30	25	20	15	10	5	0	–5	–10	–15	–20	–25	–30
CALM	*2*	*–1*	*–4*	*–7*	*–9*	*–12*	*–15*	*–18*	*–21*	*–23*	*–26*	*–29*	*–32*	*–34*

Equivalent Temperature (Fahrenheit/Centigrade)

5 MPH	33	27	21	16	12	7	1	–6	–11	–15	–20	–26	–31	–35
8 KPH	*1*	*–3*	*–6*	*–9*	*–11*	*–14*	*–17*	*–21*	*–24*	*–26*	*–29*	*–32*	*–35*	*–37*
10 MPH	21	16	9	2	–2	–9	–15	–22	–27	–31	–38	–45	–52	–58
16 KPH	*–6*	*–9*	*–13*	*–17*	*–19*	*–23*	*–26*	*–30*	*–33*	*–35*	*–39*	*–43*	*–47*	*–50*
15 MPH	16	11	1	–6	–11	–18	–25	–33	–40	–45	–51	–60	–65	–70
24 KPH	*–9*	*–12*	*–17*	*–21*	*–24*	*–28*	*–32*	*–36*	*–40*	*–43*	*–46*	*–51*	*–54*	*–57*
20 MPH	12	3	–4	–9	–17	–24	–32	–40	–46	–52	–60	–68	–76	–81
32 KPH	*–11*	*–16*	*–20*	*–23*	*–27*	*–31*	*–36*	*–40*	*–43*	*–47*	*–51*	*–56*	*–60*	*–63*
25 MPH	7	0	–7	–15	–22	–29	–37	–45	–52	–58	–67	–75	–83	–89
40 KPH	*–14*	*–18*	*–22*	*–26*	*–30*	*–34*	*–38*	*–43*	*–47*	*–50*	*–55*	*–59*	*–64*	*–67*
30 MPH	5	–2	–11	–18	–26	–33	–41	–49	–56	–63	–70	–78	–87	–94
48 KPH	*–15*	*–19*	*–24*	*–28*	*–32*	*–36*	*–41*	*–45*	*–51*	*–53*	*–57*	*–61*	*–66*	*–70*
35 MPH	3	–4	–13	–20	–27	–35	–43	–52	–60	–67	–72	–83	–90	–98
56 KPH	*–16*	*–20*	*–25*	*–31*	*–33*	*–37*	*–42*	*–47*	*–51*	*–55*	*–58*	*–64*	*–68*	*–72*
40 MPH	1	–4	–15	–22	–29	–36	–45	–54	–62	–69	–76	–87	–94	–101
64 KPH	*–17*	*–20*	*–26*	*–30*	*–34*	*–38*	*–43*	*–48*	*–52*	*–56*	*–60*	*–66*	*–70*	*–74*

Convective cooling is much greater in water than in air because the specific heat of water (the amount of heat required to warm the water) is far larger. Indeed, persons who fall into cold water lose heat less rapidly if they hold still because the convective cooling produced when the water is stirred by swimming is much greater than the heat generated by the physical activity. (See Chapter Seven, "Immersion Hypothermia.")

Conduction

Conduction is the transfer of heat energy away from the body by substances with which it is in direct contact. Air conducts heat poorly and still air, which does not cause convective heat loss, is an excellent insulator. Water has a conductivity 240 times greater than air and is a good heat conductor. Large amounts of heat are lost when the body is in contact with cold water even though movement and convective heat loss are minimized.

Stones and ice are good conductors, which explains why one's bottom gets cold when sitting on them. Metal is an excellent heat conductor. Cold metal can produce almost instant freezing of tissues which it contacts, as many who have lost skin to cold mail boxes, garbage can lids, or ice trays can attest. The ground is a good conductor, and insulation such as foam pads is required by those sleeping on the ground to minimize heat loss. Several recently developed plastic foams provide much greater comfort than older products.

Alcohol (ethanol) is a good conductor that remains liquid at temperatures well below the freezing temperature of water. A few intemperate residents of arctic climates have learned just how cold a beverage with a high alcohol content can become when they have taken a swallow from a bottle left outside or in an unheated car during winter. The extremely cold alcohol almost instantly freezes the lips, tongue, and other tissues it contacts. If the liquid reaches the back of the throat and the esophagus, the resulting injury is often lethal.

The body gains heat by conduction when in contact with hot water bottles or heating pads, or when immersed in a hot bath or a hot tub.

Evaporation

Evaporation is responsible for twenty to thirty percent of heat loss in temperate conditions. Changing one gram of water on the skin from a liquid to a gas extracts approximately 580 calories of heat, which is the reason perspiring is such an effective means of cooling.

About two-thirds of the evaporative heat loss in thermoneutral conditions occurs on the skin. In such situations the individual is not aware that he is sweating, but the skin is continually being moistened by "insensible" perspiration. Insensible perspiration continues in cold environments.

The remaining evaporative heat loss takes place in the air passages leading to the lungs. This also is an insensible water—and heat—loss. When air is inhaled, enough water is added by evaporation from the lining of the nose and throat (the mucosa) to bring the relative humidity to one hundred percent or saturation. The combined insensible water loss from the skin and respiratory tract is about thirty grams of water per hour, resulting in a heat loss of about eighteen kilocalories per hour.

Heat loss through evaporation is obviously greatly increased by the heavy sweating associated with the high heat production of vigorous exercise or a hot environment. Surprisingly, evaporative heat losses may increase in a cold environment also.

Cold air is dry. Although the relative humidity of very cold air may be high, its actual water content is low, and the relative humidity can drop to less than ten percent when the air is warmed to body temperature. However, in the air passages leading to the lungs the air is moistened to a relative humidity of almost one hundred percent, or saturation. (If it were not moistened, the very dry air would injure the lungs.) In a cold climate more heat may be lost by evaporation to humidify inhaled air than is lost by warming the air to body temperature.

At high altitudes respirations are deeper and more rapid to compensate for the "thin" air. Three to four liters of water are required each day to humidify inhaled air. The evaporation of that amount of water extracts 1,500 to 2,000 kilocalories, and also can lead to dehydration, which aggravates the effects of hypothermia.

Evaporation of water from wet clothing causes great heat loss, particularly in a wind. Wet clothing is also a threat because it loses its insulating ability, leading to greatly increased convective cooling.

Radiation

Radiation, usually by far the largest source of heat loss, consists of the direct emission or absorption of heat energy. The human body continuously radiates heat to nearby solid objects that have a cooler temperature. Little heat is radiated to air because it is a poor heat absorber, but all solid objects radiate heat to the sky when they are not absorbing heat from the sun. Most of this radiant heat is in the form of infrared radiation, and it is this radiation that allows warm bodies to be "seen" with infrared detectors.

The body also can gain large amounts of heat through radiation. The heat from the sun or a fire is radiant energy.

In a cold climate nearby solid objects are colder and radiant heat loss is larger. The rate of heat loss increases dramatically as the difference in temperature between the body and the object increases—in fact, as the fourth powers of the two temperatures. The formula for measuring such heat loss is

$$J_Q = -ek(T_a^4 - T_s^4)$$

where J_Q = heat loss, e = the emissivity of the surface, k = the Stefan-Boltzmann constant, and T_a and T_s = the temperatures of the air and the body surfaces.

The first item in the formula is the nature of the emitting surface, which emphasizes its significance: black or dark surfaces are better emittors than white or light colored surfaces.

Currently available clothing is of little benefit in reducing radiant heat loss because heat radiates from the body to the clothing and then radiates outward from the surface of the clothing. Attempts to cover clothing materials with a coating which would reflect heat back to the body have not achieved much success, although microfilaments are claimed to reduce radiant heat loss. Light colored clothing would also reduce radiant heat loss, but only to a limited extent.

Fortunately, clothing that controls convective or conductive heat losses can compensate for the increased heat loss through radiation that occurs in most cold wilderness environments.

CLOTHING TO PREVENT HEAT LOSS

The 1964 Four Inns walk clearly demonstrated that man in a severely cold environment requires clothing to prevent excessive heat loss. He can not compensate for severe cold by exercise generated heat alone. In harsher conditions, such as a blizzard, clothing alone may not provide adequate protection, and shelter of some kind may be necessary.

Clothing materials now available stop little of the body's radiant heat loss and, except for vapor barrier systems used at low temperatures, have even less effect on evaporative heat loss. To provide effective protection against cooling, particularly in a cold outdoor environment, clothing must greatly reduce or eliminate increased convective or conductive heat losses. The only effective means now available for preventing such heat loss is by maintaining immobile layers of warm air next to the body, which is the essence of insulation.

Coping With Temperature Changes

Obviously, outdoor temperatures are not constant. Cooler night and morning temperatures usually rise during the day to a maximum in midafternoon and then fall in the evening. Changes in cloud cover or the passage of a front can produce dramatic temperature changes. Additionally, heat production varies widely. Heat generation is high during vigorous activity, but falls to much lower levels during rest stops or routine activities around camp.

Clothing for a cold environment must be able to compensate for such changes in temperature and heat production. With currently available materials such compensation can best be achieved by wearing multiple layers. During warmer times of day and periods of high heat production, the outer layers must be opened or removed. When colder temperatures are encountered or energy output falls, the outer layers must be closed or additional layers added.

Although multilayered clothing systems are simple, using them effectively requires very close attention to details and usually some experience. Of particular importance is the absolute necessity for avoiding excessive sweating.

Individuals in cold environments usually dress so they remain warm while inactive. As a result, once they begin exercising they quickly start to perspire. When they cease their activity, their sweat dampened clothes have lost much of their insulation value, and the continued evaporation of moisture produces even more cooling. Outer clothing layers must be opened or taken off before sweating begins. They must be closed or put back on as soon as activity ceases, not after the individual becomes cold. If the outer layers are not opened until the individual becomes hot, sweating is unavoidable. If the outer layers are not closed until the individual feels cold, additional heat is required to warm the body again.

When removing clothing to avoid perspiring, the mittens or gloves should go first, unless protection from ice or snow is needed. Headgear and neck wrappings should follow. Then jackets should be opened at the waist and sleeves. Finally, layers of clothing should be taken off. Clothing should be replaced in the reverse sequence.

The Brynje vest or Norwegian string shirt, if properly worn, can be a valuable aid for avoiding dampening clothing with perspiration. However, the use of this unique and valuable undergarment is not widely understood. This vest should be worn next to the skin underneath the insulating clothing. As the wearer becomes warm, the outer clothing should be opened at the waist and at the neck. Cold air is warmed and expands as it comes in contact with the body at the waist. The warm air tends to rise through the chimneylike structures produced by the openings in the vest and flow out through the opening at the neck, producing a current of air over the skin of the trunk. Since the air in cold climates is relatively dry, perspiration evaporates rapidly. The result is a draft of air over the skin of the chest and upper abdomen that forcibly removes perspiration and keeps the skin and overlying clothing dry.

The Brynje vest is not an insulating garment. The openings were designed to allow air to flow freely and are too large to immobilize air, as insulation does. The vest should be made of nonabsorbent material; the originals were waxed to block water absorption.

Another essential, but commonly ignored, feature of a multilayered clothing system is the need for successive outer layers to be larger than those underneath. If the layers are the same size, the outer layers compress those underneath and eliminate much of the insulative properties. Each layer must be large enough to allow an air space one quarter inch thick between it and the layer below.

Measuring Insulation Values

Insulation is measured in "clo" units. One clo unit represents the insulation value of a typical business suit. Military polar clothing in 1966 had an insulation value of three clo units; down clothing can have values up to seven clo units. Some retailers of outdoor clothing and equipment have begun listing the clo values for insulative garments in their catalogs.

The clo unit was derived from measurements of total body insulation; one clo equals 0.18 I, which is determined by the following formula:

$$I = \frac{T_s - T_a}{H}$$

I = insulation, T_s = average skin temperature, T_a = ambient temperature, and H = heat loss from the body in kilocalories per square meter of body surface area per hour.

Insulation, "I," is derived from several sources:

$$I = I_t + I_a + I_{ce}$$

I_t = insulation value of the tissues, which is greater with a thicker layer of subcutaneous fat. I_a = insulation value of air, which is strikingly reduced by wind or when the individual is moving. I_{ce} = insulation value of the clothing being worn.

Heat, "H," also is derived from multiple sources: metabolic heat, "M"; mechanical work, "W"; evaporative heat loss from the skin and lungs, "E"; loss of stored heat, "S"; and the body surface area, "SA." Their relationships are expressed by the formula:

$$H = \frac{M - (W + E + S)}{SA}$$

Changes in Insulating Values

In experimental studies, clothing which had a clo value of 2.49 units when dry and in still air fell in value to 1.40 clo in a wind of only 2.5 mph (4 kph). With exercise, which disturbs the thin layer of air adjacent to the skin, the clo value fell to 1.04 units; wind and exercise combined to further lower the value to 0.71 units. When the wearer was active, wet, and facing a wind of 9 mph (14.5 kph), the clo value was 0.4 units—fifteen percent of its insulation value when dry and in still air! With waterproof outer garments which kept the clothing dry and protected the wearer from wind, the clo value of the clothing rose to 0.85 units, which was close to the value for dry clothing in still air during exercise.

PROTECTIVE CLOTHING

Clothing Materials

Many different materials are used for cold weather clothing. The oldest—wool—is still one of the best. Woolen fabrics contain innumerable small air pockets that provide excellent insulation. The fabric is durable and withstands wear well. One of wool's greatest values is its ability to provide insulation when wet. Even when saturated with water, wool still has about eighty percent of its dry insulation value. Wool is the material of choice for sweaters, shirts, light jackets, pants, and underwear (along with polypropylene, which is described below), particularly when a significant possibility of getting wet is present. The only major disadvantage of wool is its relatively greater weight.

Down provides excellent insulation—when it is dry. No other material provides such warmth at a comparable weight. However, when wet, down mats together and provides little insulation. Down is becoming increasingly popular, and supplies are limited. Most currently available down filled garments contain a significant percentage of feathers. (Federal Trade Commission guidelines specify that garments containing fillings labeled "down" shall contain seventy percent down clusters, ten percent down fiber, a maximum of eighteen percent feathers, and two percent residue. Fillings labled 90/10, 80/20, 70/30, or 60/40 can contain twenty-five percent, thirty-two percent, thirty-nine percent, and forty-six percent feathers.) Developing trade with China promises to make larger quantities of prime quality down available. Down is the filler of choice for sleeping bags, parkas, and overpants to be used in climates where precipitation is in the form of relatively dry snow, which is typical of high altitudes.

Polyester fibers have been developed as a substitute for down in sleeping bags and outer garments to be used in wet climates. Polyester fibers retain their loft and much of their insulation value when wet. Also, they are less expensive than down. Polyester fibers suffer the disadvantages of being heavier and much less compressible than down. Sleeping bags filled with polyester fibers occupy approximately fifty percent more space than down filled bags and are also somewhat heavier for the same amount of insulation. However, fiber manufacturers are continually improving their products, and equipment manufacturers are developing innovative designs to decrease weight and increase warmth.

Polarguard is made up of "continuous," or uncut, filaments. Their length allows them to be sewn directly to the supporting shell and makes them more durable. Other polyester fibers are shorter and more difficult to stabilize. They are more difficult to work with and therefore garments made from these fibers tend to be more expensive.

Quallofil has about twenty-five percent more loft than the other polyester fibers in its raw state, but after use, its loft advantage drops to about eight percent. This fiber has a silicone finish to reduce friction between adjacent fibers, so it feels much softer than the other resin coated polyester fibers—almost as soft as down. However, because they do not have a binding, the short fibers must be sandwiched between a double layer of film for stabilization. This film adds weight, and sleeping bags made with this fiber tend to be heavier than bags filled with other fibers. Quallofil is also more expensive than the other fibers.

Very thin polyester fibers (microfilaments) have been used for some types of clothing, particularly ski jackets and gloves. Microfilaments have a diameter of about five microns instead of the forty micron diameter of the larger filaments. These small filaments are claimed to immobilize as much air as the larger filaments in a much thinner layer because the thickness of the layer of immobilized air around the filament is the same regardless of the filament diameter. Therefore these garments are not as bulky as those made of larger filaments or down. Additionally, pads of microfilaments are claimed to reflect some radiant heat back toward the body, reducing heat loss from that source.

Microfilaments have some disadvantages. Garments containing these filaments are not as soft or bulky as garments containing larger filaments or down. They do not conform to the body surface (drape) well and allow air to circulate beneath the garment, increasing heat loss. Manufacturers must use wrist elastic or snaps, waist skirts, and snug necks to reduce this air flow. Also these materials are almost twice as heavy and much less compressible than down of equal protective value.

Garments for outdoor wear made of other artificial fibers have recently been developed. One of the most promising of these new materials is polypropylene, a polymer, or plastic, used in water bottles. When used in underwear this material transmits moisture to its surface where it can evaporate without cooling the skin. This fabric also retains much of its insulation value when wet. To take advantage of its unique moisture transmission qualities, polypropylene has been used by itself or in combination with other fibers in a variety of garments.

Polypropylene does have a few significant disadvantages. It tends to retain body odors unless vigorously laundered, and has been known to melt when dried by itself in a clothes dryer on high heat. When other garments are present in the dryer, melting is not a problem.

Fiber "pile" jackets, pants, and hats are made of polyester or nylon fibers. These garments provide insulation equivalent to a heavy wool sweater and are lighter and more durable than knitted garments. Like knitted materials, pile fabrics are porous and provide little protection from wind. The nylon fibers do not absorb water, which is a significant advantage. When wet, garments made of nylon can be wrung almost dry and put back on immediately.

Pile garments formerly offered little wind resistance and tended to "pill" or form numerous small pellets on the surface. Newly introduced pile fabrics have more wind resistance as the result of higher density, and also resist pilling to a greater degree.

Vapor Barrier Systems

Vapor barrier systems employ a layer of vapor impermeable material, usually plastic or a coated fabric, beneath a single layer or between two layers of insulation. The purpose of this barrier is to retard evaporation of moisture from insensible perspiration and thereby limit evaporative heat loss. The problem with such systems is that the moisture collects beneath the barrier. Unless such systems are used in freezing or colder temperatures at which insensible perspiration is greatly reduced, water accumulation is usually so excessive that clothing or sleeping bag liners become saturated, lose their insulative properties, and overall protection from the cold is greatly reduced. However, when used in such cold conditions, vapor barrier systems are definitely beneficial. The principal uses of vapor barrier systems at the present time are as socks and in sleeping bags. However, active development of other garments which utilize this principle is underway.

Mittens

Cold, painful toes and fingers are among the most common cold weather complaints but also are among the easiest to remedy, if the physiologic reactions to cold are kept in mind. When the body is cooled, its first response is to close down the blood vessels to the extremities to conserve heat. In contrast, when the body is warmed, the blood vessels in the extremities dilate so that more blood can flow through the skin and heat can be lost. In a cold environment, warming the body increases the blood flow to the hands and feet and keeps them warm. High quality boots and mittens are essential for protection from snow and ice, but "another sweater" does more to keep the hands and feet warm and comfortable.

Mittens can be much warmer than gloves. Human fingers are such thin cylinders that insulation thicker than one-quarter inch is ineffective. Heat is lost by radiation from the surface of protective clothing. If the area of that surface increases, heat loss increases. Inserting more than one-quarter inch of insulation into the fingers of gloves increases the surface area so much that the increased heat loss eliminates any benefits from the extra insulation. Therefore, making gloves with fingers thicker than one-quarter inch not only makes them so bulky that delicate movements are impossible, it does not increase protection from the cold.

Because mittens are so much larger than glove fingers, thicker insulation does not increase their surface area significantly and does increase their warmth.

For severe conditions the best protection seems to be provided by a three layer combination: a thin inner glove of silk or nylon, a thick middle layer of wool, down, or similar material, and an outer windproof, water repellent shell. Large, bulky mittens filled with down or polyester fibers are needed mostly in arctic climates and at very high altitudes—or for individuals who have not learned that the best way to keep the hands and feet warm is to keep the body warm.

Headgear

Three functional and anatomic features make the head and neck together a major potential source of heat loss: the blood flow to the brain is large, the bone which surrounds that organ is a good conductor of heat, and the overlying scalp is thin and contains little insulating fat. Warm headgear is an essential element of cold weather clothing. Caps made of wool or a similar insulating material are the best type of headgear currently available. The cap must cover the ears and back of the neck. The narrow knitted bands sometimes worn by skiers protect the ears, but do not significantly limit heat loss. Balaclavas, which cover the neck and most of the face, are desirable for severe conditions, particularly in strong winds.

Although hoods do cover the neck and much of the face, they are not as effective as caps for preventing heat loss because they do not fit as snugly. In severe weather a windproof and water repellent outer hood can be worn over a cap, or a down hood with a cap underneath.

Underclothing

Underclothing must maintain a layer of insulation immediately adjacent to the skin. Because underwear can be moistened by perspiration, it must retain its insulating ability when wet. Two insulating materials that are suitable for underclothing and have this property are polypropylene and wool. Polypropylene is comfortable, provides good insulation, and transmits moisture away from the skin to evaporate on the fabric's surface. Since the moisture is not evaporating on the skin surface, polypropylene underwear feels warmer. Wool is cheaper than polypropylene and possibly is somewhat warmer for its weight. Wool is thought to suffer the disadvantage of becoming "scratchy" after being washed a few times, but polypropylene, as it becomes worn, loses some of its softness also. The scratchiness of wool can be avoided by adding a small amount of oil (such as olive oil) to the rinse water to replace the natural oils removed by soap and detergents.

Raingear

In a cold climate clothing must be kept dry. Most clothing loses almost all of its insulating value when it becomes wet. In his environmental chamber investigations, physiologist Griffith Pugh studied well conditioned individuals in wet clothing at a temperature of 41° F (5° C) in a 9.4 mph (15 kph) wind. The clothing, which consisted of a string vest, wool shirt and jersey, padded parka with hood, jeans, heavy wool socks, gym shoes, and wool gloves, had an insulation value of 2.58 clo units when the wearer was dry and at rest. When the subjects were active, this wet clothing had an insulation value of only 0.39 units. A work output of 2.2 to 2.9 LO_2/min (liters of oxygen per minute; described further on page 34), which is equivalent to running at a rate of 6 mph (10 kph), was required for the subjects just to stay comfortably warm.

Garments to be worn for protection from rain should have two properties: they must keep out the rain, but they also must "breathe" or allow water vapor to escape so the wearer does not become soaked by his own perspiration. No material currently available combines these two properties in an ideal manner. Two types of fabric come close.

Laminates are made up of multiple layers of material, one of which contains innumerable pores that are large enough to allow water vapor to escape but too small to allow the larger droplets of liquid water to pass through. The best known of these laminates is Gore-Tex, which is made with a teflon film applied to the fabric. However, laminates still present some problems. They are expensive. The earlier laminates had a tendency to delaminate and could be "poisoned" by perspiration and other substances so that they no longer "breathed." Currently, Gore-Tex and garments made of Gore-Tex are being sold with a three year warranty for these problems. Considerable difficulty is still being encountered in sealing the seams. The manufacturer of Gore-Tex has a program to test the construction of garments made of that fabric. Garments that can meet their standards are given a "Raingear Without Compromise" label. Additional problems with laminates have included low resistance to abrasion, stiffness of the fabric, and noisiness, but these problems are being solved. During heavy exertion, the amount of moisture produced can exceed the capability of the laminate to transmit water vapor. Vents have been placed in some garments made of laminates so that more moisture can escape. Fabrics with an absorbent backing, which can hold the excess moisture and subsequently release it through the laminate, are also being used.

The second type of rainwear fabric either is very tightly woven so that the pores between the threads are very small, or is made of two fibers, one of which is cotton, which swells when wet and tends to close off the pores. None of the fabrics provide protection in a heavy rain, as was learned from the Four Inns disaster. Some provide little protection from the wind.

Water repellent sprays have been used to try to increase (or, for older, well worn garments, restore) water repellent qualities. Some manufacturers have resorted to completely waterproof materials or coatings and have tried to design openings that would allow perspiration to evaporate. One such garment that has been around for many years is the poncho, which can be worn so loosely that water vapor can escape below its skirt. However, with heavy exertion the wearer still gets soaked by his own perspiration.

Another lesson learned from the Four Inns tragedy was the need to protect the lower extremities from wind and water as well as the upper body. The same fabrics can be used for rain pants, although the completely impervious ones may work somewhat better because the legs do not perspire as heavily as the trunk.

Regardless of the type of fabric used, certain elements of design are essential for rainwear to be effective. The hood must close snugly enough to keep water out, but should not restrict movement of the head. The hood also must be large enough to fit over a cap or whatever headgear is being worn. Shoulder seams leak notoriously. Preferably, no seams should extend across the top of the shoulders where they can be distorted by pack straps. Dropped seams that run across the front or back of the parka or raglan sleeves that extend in one piece to the neckline are more suitable. Special care must be taken with the seams regardless of where they are located. The number of seams should be minimized, and they should be sealed with tape or by "welding." Zippers are not waterproof nor are they made of waterproof fabric. They must be covered, preferably by a waterproof flap which can be secured with snaps or Velcro. A flap behind the zipper helps prevent drafts, but is less essential than one in front. Pockets should be covered by flaps which keep water out. Cuffs should be closable with snaps or Velcro because elastic cuffs tend to ride up and can not be adjusted and knit cuffs, if not covered with waterproof material, get wet and tend to stay that way. Finally, any parka must be large enough to fit loosely and comfortably over insulating clothing that might be worn underneath.

Footgear

One of the warmest types of footgear yet devised is the U.S. Army double vapor barrier boot known as the white Korean (or Mickey Mouse) boot. This boot is composed of inner and outer rubberized layers with layers of insulation in between. Localized cold injuries essentially do not occur in persons wearing this boot.

However, this type of footwear does have significant shortcomings. First, it is soft, almost floppy, and even though crampons can be fitted, this boot is not stiff enough for kicking steps in high angle snow or for ice climbing. Secondly, the rubberized material does not "breathe" and perspiration can not evaporate. The wearer ends the day with socks saturated with water. Without care the excessive moisture can lead to maceration of the skin. The ten percent of the population with excessive sweating of the hands and feet (hyperhidrosis) often can not wear these boots. Finally, Korean boots are so costly to manufacture that they have not been made generally available. Those found in military surplus stores are either used or contain defects which have caused them to be rejected by the Army. A similar boot, which has one less layer of insulation and is colored black (the so-called black Korean boot), is available through some civilian distributors.

Excessive moisture due to sweating by wearers of vapor barrier boots or socks can be reduced sixty to seventy percent by spraying the tops of the feet with an antiperspirant. (Effective antiperspirants for the soles of the feet are not available.) An unperfumed deodorant spray or powder containing aluminum chlorhydrate or aluminum chlorhydroxide is usually cheapest and the easiest to obtain. Two or three applications a day may be necessary for about three days, but thereafter one application a day usually suffices.

Leather has long been the best material for making boots and for most uses remains the first choice. Leather can be made hard enough to protect the feet and soft enough to be flexible. It is also porous and "breathes," allowing perspiration to evaporate. For waterproofing, a material should be used which does not block these pores.

Plastic boots, which have been introduced recently, offer some definite advantages for climbers. These boots are rigid, which is essential for high angle ice climbing. Additionally, crampon straps can be cinched down tight without concern about cutting off the circulation to the feet and toes.

However, some questions have been raised about the safety of plastic boots in cold climates. The flexibility of leather boots allows them to expand slightly as the wearer's feet swell after several hours of standing or walking. (Such swelling is inevitable for anyone in an upright position.) Since plastic boots are not flexible, they can not expand to compensate for such swelling. Plastic boots are also impermeable to water vapor. Some single plastic boots have been lined with felt, which expands when wet. The combination of an inflexible plastic boot, an expanded felt liner soaked with perspiration, and swelling of the feet resulting from an upright position can compress the feet so severely that blood circulation almost ceases. Subsequent frostbite is almost unavoidable in a cold environment. Frostbite resulting from such boots has been common in the vicinity of Anchorage, Alaska.

High altitude climbing boots are usually double or triple boots. The inner boots are made of an insulating material (which would be expected to accommodate swelling of the feet.) The outer boots most often have been made of leather, but plastic outer boots have been introduced in recent years. However, a recent compilation of the incidents of frostbite on Mount McKinley has disclosed that wearers of plastic boots developed frostbite more commonly than wearers of leather boots, regardless of climbing experience or the difficulty of the routes. Perhaps the inflexibility of the plastic boots leads to significant compression of the feet in spite of the interposition of one or more insulating boots. Impermeability to water vapor may also play a role in the development of such injuries.

Hiking boots and rock climbing boots with tops of heavy fabric have recently been developed, in part because leather has become so expensive. These boots are cooler and keep the feet drier, and for many uses are entirely satisfactory. They are not intended for severe cold conditions.

Socks are largely a matter of personal choice. Many experienced outdoorsmen prefer an inner thin sock of silk, nylon, or even lightweight wool, and an outer bulky sock. This combination is useful for reducing friction that can cause blisters, but is not much warmer than a single bulky sock. For warmth, some winter outdoorsmen like to wear a vapor impermeable plastic sock between two wool socks, but this creates problems with perspiration just as vapor barrier boots do.

Regardless of the combination chosen, socks of the same thickness should be worn at all times. Adding extra socks because the weather is colder is an excellent way to ensure that boots are too tight, blood circulation is compromised, and the risk of frostbite is greatly increased. Wearing thinner socks leaves the boots too loose and tends to cause blisters.

Gaiters and overboots keep snow out of the top of the boot, which helps avoid wetting and cooling the feet. (In dry climates gaiters keep dirt, sand, or small stones out of the boots.) Some gaiters and overboots have a lining of insulating material such as ensolite or felt, which does help keep the feet warm in severe conditions.

Other garments

The selection of shirts, sweaters, jackets, parkas, pants, or overpants will depend upon the climatic conditions anticipated. Shirts which cover the neck, such as those with "turtle necks," are more comfortable in cold weather, but can not be opened when the wearer becomes warm. The long established value of a wool scarf should not be ignored.

Regardless of the garments worn or the materials of which they are made, intelligent use of the clothing is still the most essential element for protection from cold.

SHELTER

A full discussion of shelters for cold weather protection, particularly techniques for constructing such shelters, is beyond the scope of this publication. However, a brief consideration of the essential features of shelters for preventing cold injuries does seem appropriate.

In a cold climate temporary shelters, including tents, must provide protection from the convective cooling of wind. Tents are not windproof and in severe conditions usually require some kind of windbreak. Snow shelters, such as caves, igloos, or just a hole dug in the snow and covered with a tarp, tent, or tree limbs, are much more effective than tents. Such shelters completely block the wind and eliminate severe convective cooling. Additionally, since the air inside is relatively stationary, it can be warmed by heat from the body and provide a much more comfortable environment. If a large cave or hole is dug where wood is available, a fire can be built to provide warmth.

Shelter must also provide protection from moisture and conductive cooling. Tent floors and lower walls must be waterproof. The upper portion of the tent must "breathe" so the moisture (and the carbon dioxide) in exhaled air can escape. At temperatures below freezing, the moisture in exhaled air tends to collect on tent walls, freeze, and drop down on the sleepers below. It may be melted by their body heat and tend to dampen the outer surface of their sleeping bags. No completely adequate solution for this problem is available. Snow shelters "breathe" adequately, but some protection from snow melted by the body when sitting or lying on its surface is essential. An insulating pad is best; a tarp or similar waterproof material is better than nothing.

HEAT PRODUCTION

Heat Generated by Exercise

Heat production by the body can be increased significantly only by muscular exercise, either by shivering or by voluntary work directed toward a specific goal (such as getting out of a cold environment.) The large muscles in the legs can produce more heat than smaller muscles. Vigorously exercising those large muscles also can produce more heat than shivering. If a threatening situation can not be escaped—which clearly would be the most desirable type of voluntary heat producing exercise—deliberate exercise that utilizes those large muscles, such as repeatedly stepping up onto and off of rocks or logs, produces more heat than just standing around shivering.

No drugs or other behavior can substitute for exercise as a means for generating heat.

Food Metabolism

If the body is to generate heat, food must be absorbed and converted into compounds which can be metabolized. These compounds are composed of carbon and hydrogen, which must be combined with oxygen in a series of complex biochemical reactions to form carbon dioxide and water. During these reactions, heat is produced and additional energy is stored in chemical bonds to be released in the performance of chemical or mechanical work.

In a resting state, all of the energy from metabolism ultimately becomes heat. During physical activity, including vigorous exercise, only about twenty percent of this chemical energy is used for mechanical work. The other eighty percent is converted into heat. However, the quantity of heat resulting from physical activity is far greater than 100 percent of the heat produced in the resting state.

Energy from the metabolism of food is usually measured in kilocalories. One kilocalorie equals one thousand ordinary calories. Confusion arises because in common usage kilocalories are referred to as calories. That chocolate cream pie which contains 500 calories per bite actually contains 500,000 calories or 500 kilocalories per bite. To avoid confusion, kilocalories are sometimes referred to as "large" calories and are abbreviated "Cal" with a capital "c" or "kcal." However, this convention is used quite inconsistently.

Generally speaking, metabolism of one gram of carbohydrate yields four calories, metabolism of one gram of fat yields nine calories, and metabolism of one gram of protein yields a little less than four calories. Although a high fat diet would contain more calories and could be more useful for situations demanding a high caloric expenditure, such as high altitude mountaineering, such diets are unpalatable. A balanced diet, with equal amounts of all three types of food, is more acceptable; some people prefer a high carbohydrate diet. For prolonged outings a balanced diet is needed to provide adequate noncaloric nutrition.

In contemporary Western societies most individuals require approximately 1,800 to 3,000 kilocalories per day, depending upon their body size and how much physical work they do. Individuals who are very active may require much more.

Glucose is by far the major source of metabolic energy for exercising muscles. Glucose is present in the blood, but is stored in muscles—and in much larger quantities in the liver—largely as glycogen. These stores are limited. They are adequate for only a few hours of exercise and then have to be replaced. (Conditioning can increase glycogen stores to some extent.)

The only source of glucose to rapidly replace that which has been metabolized is food. (The body's fat is a major source of energy—sometimes a huge source of energy—but fat cannot be mobilized and metabolized fast enough to serve as an energy source during vigorous exercise.) Anyone depending upon exercise generated heat to avoid hypothermia must consume large quantities of food.

The Four Inns hikers were estimated to have had an energy output equivalent to 6,000 kilocalories. Their average intake of only 1,000 to 1,500 kilocalories was a major contributor to the high incidence of hypothermia.

Consuming enough food in the conventional three or four daily meals to provide the extra calories needed for vigorous physical activity and for preventing hypothermia presents problems in a wilderness situation. Preparing the meals requires too much time. Furthermore, experienced outdoorsmen have found the best means for maintaining an adequate food intake to be repeated small snacks. Some seem to be almost continuously nibbling—but they rarely become hypothermic! A variety of trail foods, often referred to as "gorp," has been developed to simplify this type of continuous consumption. Each wilderness user must find the type of food and pattern for eating which best fits his individual tastes. However, a high food intake is an essential element of any effort to avoid hypothermia.

Oxygen Consumption during Hypothermia

The oxygen consumption for a given level of work is greatly increased when the body core temperature has fallen below normal. Since oxygen is used to metabolize food, heat production can be measured conveniently in terms of the amount of oxygen consumed in the process. The value is most commonly expressed as liters of oxygen consumed per minute (LO_2/min). Much of the data gathered during experimental studies of hypothermia has been expressed in terms of oxygen consumption. Understanding the significance of different oxygen consumption rates is essential for understanding the results of those investigations.

When resting, a typical healthy man consumes 0.25 to 0.33 LO_2/min. Walking on level ground at three miles per hour increases oxygen consumption to about 1.1 L/min. Young climbers in good physical condition habitually work at oxygen consumption rates of 2.0 to 2.5 L/min, which is sixty to seventy percent of their capacity.

Climbing members of the British 1953 Mount Everest expedition generally worked at oxygen consumption rates of 1.45 to 1.98 L/min. Their maximal oxygen consumption ranged from about 2.0 to 3.75 L/min. (Interestingly, the Sherpas had maximal oxygen consumptions of only about 2.2 to 2.7 L/min.) International class distance runners can achieve oxygen consumption rates as high as 5.0 L/min.

Expressed another way, an oxygen consumption of 2.5 L/min is equivalent to the production of about 600 kilocalories per hour. About 100 kilocalories are expended in walking or running one mile on level ground regardless of speed, so the expenditure of 600 kilocalories per hour would be equivalent to walking six miles per hour or a rate of ten minutes per mile. Only well conditioned individuals can maintain such an exercise level for very long; no one can keep it up indefinitely. An oxygen uptake of 5 L/min is comparable to travelling twelve miles per hour. The world's best marathoners can maintain that level of energy output for only a little over two hours. Pugh used a specially designed environmental chamber to demonstrate that resting individuals had a dramatic increase in oxygen consumption (from an average of 0.28 L/min to 1.02 L/min) after a body temperature drop of only 1.1° F (0.62° C). Their oxygen consumption increased 360 percent with no visible work being performed! Although lying quietly, they were consuming as much oxygen as they would have while walking at a rate of three miles per hour when normothermic. Subjects whose temperatures had fallen 0.9° to 1.8° F (0.5° to 1.0° C) required an additional 0.4 to 0.5 LO_2/min to perform work carried out at oxygen consumption rates of 1.1 to 1.6 L/min by persons with normal body temperatures, an increase ranging from twenty-five to fifty percent.

Pugh found that hikers spontaneously increased their work output to maintain a normal core temperature whenever their skin temperature fell below comfortable levels (84° to 88°F or 29° to 31°C). For some hikers the resulting pace produced exhaustion and near collapse.

These findings sound a clear warning for outdoorsmen. Since even mildly hypothermic individuals have to expend much more energy than normothermic persons to perform the same amount of work, those who are not in top physical condition may not be able to maintain such energy expenditure levels long enough to restore normal temperature, or to hike out of a threatening situation. Once such individuals became hypothermic, they would be unable to escape without a major change in their circumstances! That major change would have to be in the form of abundant extra clothing, shelter, or an external source of heat such as a fire, because they would be unable to generate sufficient heat to rewarm themselves by exercise.

Clearly, hypothermia should be avoided, not treated.

ADDITIONAL READING

Adolph EF, Molna GW: Exchanges of heat and tolerances to cold in men exposed to outdoor weather. *Amer J Physiol* 1946;146:507-37.

Freeman J, Pugh LGCE: Hypothermia in mountain accidents. *Internat Anesth Clinic* 1969;7:997-1007.

Hervey GR: Hypothermia. *Proc Roy Soc Med* 1973;66:1053-7.

Maclean D, Emslie-Smith D: *Accidental Hypothermia.* Oxford: Blackwell Scientific Publications, 1977.

Pugh, LGCE: Muscular exercise on Mount Everest. *J Physiol* 1958;141:233-61.

Pugh, LGCE: Clothing insulation and accidental hypothermia in youth. *Nature* 1966;209:1281-6.

Pugh, LGCE: Cold stress and muscular exercise, with special reference to accidental hypothermia. *Brit Med J* 1967;2:333-7.

CHAPTER THREE

Responses to Cooling

CAMERON C. BANGS, M.D.

Preventing, recognizing, or treating cold injuries requires an understanding of the effects of cold on the body. Romantics might object to considering all human functions to be the end results of millions and millions of biochemical reactions, but that concept is not inappropriate. An appreciation of the effects of cooling requires such a cold hearted approach. All biochemical reactions require a certain amount of time for completion; the time is always prolonged if the reactants are cooled. Biochemical reactions have an optimal temperature, which for those occurring in humans is the normal body temperature. The efficiency of the reactions and the manner in which they mesh with other biochemical reactions is disturbed by temperatures which are higher or lower than normal. As the body is cooled, all functions become slower and less efficient, although such slowing often is not noticeable until cooling is rather severe.

Solutions tend to increase in viscosity, or thicken, as they are cooled. Like automobile engine oil on a cold morning or cold maple syrup poured over pancakes, blood also thickens when cooled. Pliable materials such as plastics become stiff and rigid when cooled. Muscles do also.

The molecules in gases bounce off one another less vigorously when cooled, which allows them to come closer together and occupy a smaller volume and increases their solubility in liquids. The increased solubility of oxygen in the cold blood of the ice fish allows all of the oxygen needed for that animal's metabolism to be carried in solution. That species does not need—and does not have—hemoglobin to carry oxygen.

The body is composed of a number of separate organ systems,

each of which must function effectively if all are to survive. For example, the circulatory system carries nutrients digested and absorbed by the gastrointestinal system to the liver, where they may be further modified. The nutrients are then carried to muscles, where they are broken down into water and carbon dioxide. The circulation carries the excess water to the kidneys, where it is eliminated, and the carbon dioxide to the lungs, where it is exhaled.

Cold does not affect all organ systems uniformly. But it can cause one system to fail, which in turn causes others to fail.

Until the core temperature approaches 90° F (32° C) the body's response to cooling consists mostly of efforts to restore normal temperature. (See Chapter One, "The Control of Body Temperature.") In general, as the body begins to cool, all systems are impaired equally, and the effects tend to balance one another. For example, cooling slows the chemical reactions requiring oxygen. As a result, the metabolic need for oxygen diminishes in proportion to the reduced supply from the lungs and circulatory systems. With profound hypothermia, the changes in function become more abnormal and are often deleterious to the body as a whole. The reduction in oxygen supply is usually greater than the reduction in oxygen demand.

With few exceptions, the physiologic changes induced by rapid cooling by immersion in cold water differ very little from those caused by slower cooling in air. Water immersion may be complicated by water in the lungs or near drowning. Slower cooling in air allows more time for undesirable metabolic changes, which can hinder or totally prevent the victim's recovery.

CHANGES IN SPECIFIC ORGANS

Muscles

Mild cooling causes muscle stiffness and incoordination by directly affecting the muscle tissue. The amount of oxygen consumed in the performance of simple tasks increases tremendously (See Chapter Two, "Avoiding Hypothermia.") Involuntary shivering causes some incoordination, but that can be overcome by voluntary movement. Profound cooling causes an actual decrease in the rate at which nerve impulses are conducted to the muscles, as well as a decrease in the response by the muscle tissue. As a result the muscles are unable to contract effectively (weakness), and contracted muscles may be unable to relax (tetany). The result is jerky, uncoordinated movements, staggering, and loss of the ability to perform even simple tasks, such as zipping up a jacket. Victims of prolonged cold water immersion may be unable to assist in their rescue.

Shivering usually tapers off or ceases as body temperatures fall below 90° F (32° C), leading to a decrease in heat production. Violent shivering can lead to the metabolic production of acids, which accumulate in the blood and cause it to become more acid, a condition known as "acidosis." Shivering can also deplete the muscles of glycogen or glucose, which are necessary sources of energy for continued muscular activity—including shivering.

Brain

With mild core cooling, thinking processes and decision making become slower. Personalities become apathetic and disagreeable. However, such individuals should remain oriented and able to make correct decisions.

With profound hypothermia, mental function is impaired to a far greater extent, leading to confusion, disorientation, and erroneous decision making. The desire or ability to obtain protection from the cold is progressively lost, leading to more rapid loss of body heat. Victims of extreme hypothermia commonly take off their clothing (paradoxical disrobing). Lethargy and somnolence progress in a waxing and waning manner to complete coma. Slurred speech and loss of vision are reported to occur just prior to terminal coma.

Hypothermia markedly decreases the brain's need for oxygen. A normothermic person suffers irreversible damage if the brain is deprived of blood and the oxygen it carries for more than four or five minutes. When the brain is cold, it can tolerate a much longer time without oxygen before permanent damage occurs. This reduced need for oxygen by a hypothermic brain partially explains the occasional resuscitation without brain damage of persons (mostly children) who have been submerged in cold water for more than half an hour.

Circulatory System

The primary function of the circulatory system, which consists of the heart and the blood vessels, is to transport blood. In turn, blood carries oxygen to the tissues and carbon dioxide away from them. One of the most devastating effects of profound hypothermia is a reduction in the volume of circulating blood. This reduction can be large enough to decrease blood flow and oxygen transport to a quantity well below that needed for normal function. Vital organs such as the brain and heart, when not adequately perfused with oxygenated blood, can not perform properly, which compounds the hypothermic situation.

Because their water losses exceed their water intake, essentially all hypothermia victims are dehydrated and have a reduced blood volume. Most hypothermic individuals are unable to obtain fluids, whether they are lying in a snow bank or immobilized by senility in a cold apartment. The longer the cold exposure, the longer the period of inadequate fluid intake.

Hypothermia also increases fluid loss by producing "cold diuresis," the increased excretion of water by the kidneys. Cold diuresis is a complex phenomenon. Lying in one position for a long time increases urine flow. If a person is submerged in water, the pressure of the water on the skin squeezes fluid back into the body core. Intense constriction of blood vessels in the arms and legs, an attempt by the body to reduce heat loss in response to cooling, also forces blood back into the core. The body interprets this increased core blood volume as an indication that the body has retained too much fluid and decreases the production of antidiuretic hormone. This hormone causes the kidneys to conserve water, so a decrease in this hormone increases water loss through the kidneys. Finally, cold and insufficient oxygen directly affect the kidneys, decreasing their ability to conserve water and producing a larger urinary output.

The circulating blood volume is further decreased when the body is cooled because water leaves the circulating blood and is sequestered in the tissues. The viscosity of the blood can be increased as much as 175 percent of normal by the loss of fluid (hemoconcentration) and the direct effect of cold on the blood. Finally, cold induces contraction of the spleen, which increases the number of circulating red blood cells and thereby the blood viscosity.

As the result of decreased fluid intake, increased fluid losses, and redistribution of the fluid present, victims of several day's exposure to cold commonly have circulating blood volumes that have been reduced as much as twenty-five percent. An adequate water intake during cold exposure is absolutely essential.

Two additional changes decrease the transport of oxygen to the tissues. First, cold causes the blood vessels to constrict, reducing their diameter and increasing the resistance to flow. Second, most of the oxygen carried in the blood is bound to hemoglobin within the red blood cells. At the tissues hemoglobin normally releases oxygen, but cold hemoglobin releases its oxygen much less readily. As a result, less oxygen is actually delivered to the tissues. This diminished oxygen delivery is partially offset by two changes. First, the quantity of oxygen dissolved in the aqueous part of the blood (not carried by the hemoglobin in red blood cells) increases as it cools. At 86° F (30° C) the quantity of dissolved oxygen is nineteen percent greater than at normal body temperature. Second, the acidosis usually present increases the rate of oxygen release by hemoglobin.

Heart

At normal body temperatures the heart can force viscous blood through smaller vessels by pumping harder and faster. Unfortunately, the heart cooled to the level of profound hypothermia pumps weakly and slowly. At such temperatures the heart muscle becomes stiff and weak, and the volume of blood pumped with each beat (the stroke volume) is markedly decreased.

As the body cools to such levels, the rate of impulse conduction through the nerves and special conductive tissue that control the heart becomes slower, and the number of beats per minute falls. With deep hypothermia the heart rate may slow to as little as twenty or less per minute. Conduction also becomes erratic, contributing to irregularities of the heart beat, such as extra beats or atrial fibrillation, which reduce cardiac output (the volume of blood pumped by the heart), or ventricular fibrillation, which stops cardiac output entirely. The muscle fibers of the heart must contract almost simultaneously in a well coordinated sequence to pump blood. Ventricular fibrillation is a condition in which the individual muscle fibers contract rapidly in a totally unsynchronized, uncoordinated manner. The fibrillating heart does not pump blood. Such an event, untreated, is lethal within two or three minutes, although external cardiac compression (CPR) can keep some blood circulating for a longer time. The only treatment for ventricular fibrillation currently available is to electrically shock the heart and temporarily stop all of the fibers from contracting, hoping that when they begin contracting again they will contract in a coordinated manner. Sometimes it works, although rarely if the victim is severely hypothermic.

A hypothermic heart is particularly susceptible to ventricular fibrillation. Many minor irritants fully tolerated by the heart at normal temperatures cause a hypothermic heart to fibrillate. Once a cold heart fibrillates, restoring a normal rhythm with electrical shock is very difficult.

Some evidence suggests that when an individual dies of hypothermia before he is found—frozen in a snow bank; rescued tomorrow—his heart simply beats more and more slowly until it stops. However, an individual in profound hypothermia who dies after he has been rescued usually dies of ventricular fibrillation. His death should be considered to have been induced by the rescue or treatment—at least in part. More specific causes of ventricular fibrillation, and their avoidance, are discussed in Chapter Five, "Treatment of Hypothermia."

A slow, weak heart pumping a reduced volume of thick, viscous blood, which releases oxygen less readily, through narrowed blood vessels, can not provide the tissues with an adequate oxygen supply. Yet for the tissues to metabolize nutrients completely oxygen is essential. Without adequate oxygen metabolism is incomplete. The products of incomplete metabolism are acids, such as lactic and pyruvic acid. The accumulation of these acids in the tissues and in the blood causes acidosis (an increased hydrogen ion concentration, or a lower pH), which also causes the heart to contract more weakly and erratically.

With all of the "disasters" occurring within the cardiovascular system, the profound hypothermia victim's blood pressure could certainly be expected to be low. Surprisingly, it is usually normal or nearly normal, although occasional victims do have a low blood pressure. The reason the blood pressure remains at normal levels is probably the intense constriction of peripheral blood vessels, which increases the resistance to blood flow and keeps the pressure up. The blood pressure may be very hard to measure with a standard cuff and stethoscope because the diminished blood flow decreases the sounds by which pressure is measured.

Lungs

The effects of hypothermia on the function of the lungs has not been as well studied as the effects on the heart and circulation. Ventilation, the movement of air into and out of the lungs, is known to be adequate until core temperature drops to 90° F (32° C). At that temperature and below, carbon dioxide accumulates in the blood, indicating that ventilation is inadequate. Acidosis resulting from the accumulation of acidic metabolites is normally partially counterbalanced by increased ventilation. With profound hypothermia such respiratory compensation does not occur.

At normal body temperatures, the slight rise in carbon dioxide between breaths stimulates the brain to make the lungs take another breath and get rid of the carbon dioxide. With profound hypothermia, the brain—more specifically, the medullary respiratory centers—becomes unresponsive to carbon dioxide accumulation. The drive to breathe then derives from other sensors which are stimulated by low oxygen concentrations (hypoxia). Theoretically at least, treating hypothermia victims with oxygen could raise the blood concentration of oxygen to such levels that the hypoxic respiratory center would no longer be stimulated and the drive to breathe would be significantly reduced. Although the victim might not be hypoxic, he would accumulate more carbon dioxide, which would further increase his acidosis.

Hypothermia may increase mucus secretion by the membranes lining the trachea and bronchi, the major air passages. The cough reflex may also be decreased, allowing the excessive mucus to collect within the passages. Additionally, stomach contents may be vomited and aspirated. Either of these events often leads to a severe infection. During rewarming, the lungs may fill with fluid (pulmonary edema). Autopsies of hypothermia victims invariably disclose lung abnormalities, which include infection (pneumonia), breakdown of the small air sacs (alveoli), bleeding, and fluid accumulation (edema).

Others

Cooling the liver, as with other organs, slows its metabolic functions, but such slowing has not caused any significant problems except with drug metabolism occuring in the liver. Any medication given to a hypothermic individual is metabolized more slowly, and its effects may last much longer. Giving drugs at intervals intended for normothermic individuals may lead to an overdose. For this reason, drugs must be given cautiously or not at all during the treatment of hypothermia.

After profound hypothermia, acute pancreatitis, a serious medical complication in which the pancreas becomes inflamed and is often partially destroyed, occurs with some frequency. Additionally, the effectiveness of insulin is blunted, perhaps as the result of inadequate release by the pancreas combined with reduced activity in the tissues due to the lower temperature. Increased blood sugar concentrations are not uncommon in hypothermia victims, including those who are not diabetic.

The adrenal and thyroid glands seem to function well when cold, as evidenced by adequate concentrations of their hormones in the blood . The stomach may be affected by the stress, leading to ulcers, which occasionally cause significant bleeding. No typical changes occur in the blood sodium, potassium, or chloride concentrations.

Complications

In spite of the many pathologic changes occurring with hypothermia, hypothermia alone causes no permanent problems. All of the changes are completely reversible. No evidence indicates that hypothermia victims are subsequently more susceptible to hypothermia or less tolerant of cold.

The many complications occurring most commonly after rewarming are listed in Table 2. However, for previously healthy hypothermia victims, the risk of serious complications is low. Many of the complications result from preexisting, predisposing conditions, such as chronic alcoholism, malnutrition, or chronic debilitating diseases.

Table 2. Complications of Profound Hypothermia

1. Pneumonia
2. Acute pancreatitis
3. Intravascular clots (thromboses) causing myocardial infarcts and strokes
4. Pulmonary edema
5. Acute renal failure due to tubular necrosis
6. Increased renal potassium excretion leading to alkalosis
7. Hemolysis (breakdown of red blood cells)
8. Depressed bone marrow function
9. Inadequate blood clotting or disseminated intravascular coagulation
10. Low serum phosphorus
11. Seizures
12. Hematuria (blood in the urine)
13. Myoglobinuria (muscle pigment resembling hemoglobin in the urine)
14. Simian deformity of the hand
15. Temporary Adrenal Insufficiency
16. Gastric erosion or ulceration and bleeding

CHAPTER FOUR

Recognizing Hypothermia

CAMERON C. BANGS, M.D.

If a hiker were found frozen in a block of ice, hypothermia would certainly be suspected to have played a role in his death. If this disorder were always so obvious, its diagnosis would be simple— and unimportant. Fortunately, most victims of hypothermia do not have such a dire outcome. Unfortunately, recognizing the condition is rarely so straightforward. Most patients have only vague complaints and minimal physical abnormalities, causing hypothermia often to go unrecognized—in the mountains, along hiking trails, and in major hospital emergency rooms.

The diagnosis is important. Failure to recognize and treat hypothermia can have devastating consequences. Mild hypothermia can progress to profound hypothermia. Without proper management, profound hypothermia may be lethal.

SITUATIONS PROMOTING HYPOTHERMIA

When bullets are flying about and someone is hurt, a bullet wound is usually the cause. The same logic applies to hypothermia, although the "bullets" are much more subtle. With experience, a pattern emerges from the various situations in which hypothermia occurs. Awareness of these patterns and understanding the situations help the wary to ensure that hypothermia is not overlooked.

Urban Hypothermia
Surprisingly, hypothermia occurs more commonly in urban environments than in the wilderness. Both the very young and the very

old are more susceptible. The elderly produce less heat because they have a smaller muscle mass and often suffer from malnutrition and debilitating diseases. Medications for chronic diseases may increase heat loss by increasing the blood flow to the skin or may decrease heat production by interfering with muscle activity, particularly shivering. Poverty can cause malnutrition and may prohibit adequate heating of living quarters. A room temperature of 60° F (16° C) may be inadequate to prevent chronic body heat loss in the elderly.

The very young are more susceptible to hypothermia because they have a proportionally much greater body surface area from which heat loss occurs. Also, their temperature regulatory system is less well developed. In any given cold situation, children can be expected to cool faster. The younger the child, the more rapid the cooling.

Chronic alcoholics constitute a segment of the urban population with the highest incidence of hypothermia. Excess alcohol decreases heat production by interfering with shivering. For many chronic alcoholics poor nutrition also interferes with heat production. Heat loss is increased because alcohol dilates the blood vessels in the skin. The most important cause of hypothermia in alcoholics however, is the dumb things drunks do, such as falling asleep (passing out) outdoors or falling into water.

Immersion

Anyone in water colder than 60° to 70° F (16° to 21° C) is a prime candidate for hypothermia. Prolonged immersion in water as warm as 77° F (25° C) cools the body. However, though falling into icy water must be among the world's most miserable experiences, even ice water takes about fifteen minutes to cool the body to a level at which the individual is physically impaired. Panicky overreactions are unjustifiable and must be avoided.

Immersion cools the body fastest when the victim has no flotation device, has no protective gear or clothing, is swimming or struggling, has little body fat, is young, and is small in stature. Furthermore, a person can continue to cool after rescue if he remains in wet clothing. (See Chapter Six, "Immersion Hypothermia.")

Injuries

Injured persons cool faster than uninjured ones, particularly when they have head injuries or are in shock. The victims of such accidents may lose the ability to shiver and to constrict peripheral blood vessels. In many situations in which an uninjured person would remain warm, an injured individual rapidly becomes hypothermic.

Immobilization

A mobile person may walk for hours or even days in a cold environment without becoming hypothermic because he produces enough heat to keep warm. If the same individual is involuntarily immobilized by injuries, terrain, weather, or fatigue—or voluntarily while climbing, hunting, or fishing—heat production decreases and body temperature may drop.

Weather

The three components of weather which affect cooling most are temperature, wind, and moisture. These elements must be evaluated together, because no single one determines the effect of the weather. A person might well survive longer at 10° F (-12° C) in still, dry air, than at 40° F (4° C) when exposed to rain and high winds. (See Chapter Two, "Avoiding Hypothermia.")

Clothing and Shelter

The protection from weather offered by clothing depends upon its insulation value, which in turn depends upon the material of which it is made, its thickness, its ability to repel wind and water, and possibly its insulating ability when wet. The area of the body covered is also significant. Preventing heat loss from the head, neck, and trunk is vital.

Shelter should provide protection from wind and rain or moisture and insulation from the ground. A fire can be an invaluable source of warmth. (See Chapter Two, "Avoiding Hypothermia.")

Personal Factors

One hundred people dropped into identical life-threatening cold situations would have greatly varying survival times. Not all the reasons for this variability are known, but some patterns do seem to prolong survival. Persons who have previously experienced severe cold definitely do better when again confronted with such situations. Perhaps they do all the little things to reduce heat loss more instinctively. The ability to obtain drinking water without eating snow or ice is very important. Though food is of less immediate importance than water, food is essential for survival for more than a few days. Food is also required for vigorous exercise. Aerobic fitness delays fatigue and prolongs shivering, although the single situation when obesity can be an advantage is in the cold. Short fat people stay warmer longer than tall skinny people. Psychological stability helps to prevent emotional extremes such as giving up and not taking the protective measures that are possible, or panic that wastes energy and promotes heat loss.

EVALUATING THE HYPOTHERMIA VICTIM

No single sign or symptom except a measured low body temperature is diagnostic of hypothermia. Almost all of the changes are subtle and can be mimicked by other diseases.

After hypothermia has been diagnosed, a distinction between mild or profound (severe) hypothermia must be made. From the standpoint of caring for their victims, mild and profound hypothermia are two almost entirely different problems. The treatment of profound hypothermia (generally a temperature of 90° F [32° C] or below) is a medical emergency demanding immediate, intensive care.

Temperature Measurement

Actually measuring the body temperature is the only definitive way of documenting hypothermia. The thermometer used must be capable of recording hypothermic temperatures. (Most clinical thermometers only go down to about 93° F [34° C]). Any rescue group operating in a cold environment should carry such thermometers. However, most parties encountering victims of hypothermia are not rescue groups but are on outings for their own enjoyment. They are rarely equipped with clinical thermometers of any type and must determine the victim's level of hypothermia from the signs and symptoms he presents. (Temperature measurements are discussed more completely in Chapter One, "Control of Body Temperature.")

Mild Hypothermia

Mild hypothermia must be recognized so that rewarming can be initiated and profound hypothermia can be prevented. Typically—and fairly commonly—one or more members of a party becomes hypothermic while continuing to hike, climb, sail, ski, or whatever the group's activity. That person complains of feeling cold, often is wet, and usually is shivering to some extent, although shivering may be inapparent while he is walking. He loses interest in any activity except getting warm and often develops a negative attitude towards the group's original goals. As cooling continues he begins to develop problems with muscular coordination, usually first manifested by clumsiness with precise hand movements. Among hikers the first signs of hypothermia are inability to keep up with the rest of the party and difficulty walking over rough terrain. Later, stumbling or clumsiness with any physical task appears.

Profound Hypothermia

Profound hypothermia, which is defined as a core temperature of 90° F (32° C) or below, is characterized by altered mental function. Probably the most important tip-off that a person has become profoundly hypothermic is carelessness about protecting against the cold. Jackets are left unzipped, hoods are not pulled up, caps are not snugged down around the ears, mittens or gloves are not worn, blankets or sleeping bags are not pulled up around the neck or head, and fires are left unattended.

When a person is not doing all he can to stay warm, profound hypothermia must be suspected. Other definite, although sometimes subtle, mental changes occur at this temperature. Thinking is slow. Decision making is difficult and often erroneous. Memory for specific facts, such as dates, numbers, or names, deteriorates. The victim may have a strong desire to escape the cold by sleeping. He has lapses in his willingness to struggle for survival. Eventually, periods of unresponsiveness alternate with periods of activity. Gradually, the periods of unconsciousness become prolonged until the victim lapses into coma from which he can not be aroused. Incoherent speech and loss of vision are late events, preceding complete coma or death by a few minutes to an hour.

One abnormal behavior pattern that appears to be specific for profound hypothermia is the victim who appears to be able to cooperate but does not do so. Such actions can be quite irritating for rescuers who do not recognize this sign of hypothermia. In a number of instances, hypothermic individuals who seemed to be acting quite sensibly have made gross errors in judgement that aggravated problems for the entire party.

At profoundly hypothermic body temperatures, muscle function progressively deteriorates along with mental function. Shivering generally decreases and eventually disappears at about 90° F (32° C), although individuals vary greatly in the amount they shiver and the core temperatures at which shivering begins and ceases. Difficulty walking progresses to difficulty standing and finally the inability to do either.

Careful examination of the victim may reveal some abnormalities, but the absence of such findings should not preclude the diagnosis of profound hypothermia. The skin may feel cold and nonpliable. It may be pale and have a slight bluish hue. Evidence of frostbite, bruises, or other injuries may be present. The pupils of the eyes do not undergo any characteristic changes. The pulse is often weak and hard to feel. The pulse rate is typically slow and irregular. The blood pressure is difficult to measure and may be normal or low. Heart sounds, whether heard with the unaided ear or with a stethoscope, may be diminished in intensity. Breathing is slow and shallow. The lung sounds are usually clear, but may be harsh, rattling, or bubbling due to fluid in the lungs. The abdomen presents no typical changes.

The victim's breath frequently has a fruity, acetone odor resulting from the incomplete metabolism of fats caused by the inadequate blood supply to the peripheral tissues. This characteristic odor may be the first clue to the severity of the hypothermia. The clothing may be soaked with urine, which also indicates a serious situation.

Table 3. Most Common and Most Obvious
Findings with Profound Hypothermia

1. Mental changes, including failure to seek protection from the cold
2. Incoordination
3. Cold skin
4. Fruity acetone breath
5. Urine soaked clothing

A careful search for other injuries must be carried out according to a definite, previously established routine, as with all accident victims.

Near Death

Some victims of profound hypothermia undoubtedly have been pronounced dead and abandoned while they were still alive. A few may even have been autopsied!

Profound hypothermia can closely mimic death. The victim may appear stiff and frozen in the fetal position with legs and arms which can not be straightened. Pupils may not contract when exposed to light. Eyes may appear glassy. Pulse and respiration may be so slow and weak they can not be detected. An electrocardiogram may be required to detect any heart activity. Victims of such profound hypothermia must not be denied careful rewarming as if they were known to be alive.

At a recent international conference on cold injuries many controversial subjects and ideas were discussed. The one concept with which everyone agreed was that no one should be pronounced dead from hypothermia until his body has been warmed to near normal temperature.

No one should be considered cold and dead until he has been warm and dead!

CHAPTER FIVE

Treating Hypothermia

CAMERON C. BANGS, M.D.

No previously healthy person should die of hypothermia after he has been rescued and treatment has been started.

A bold statement, but one that should be true. The current understanding of the treatment for hypothermia is far from complete. However, enough is known for death to be avoidable for all but a very few—perhaps none—if that knowledge is properly applied after rescue. (Many urban hypothermia victims are either suffering from severe illnesses of other types or are chronic alcoholics and would not be considered "previously healthy.")

If a person has a virus infection on a business trip to New York, on a mountaineering expedition to Nepal, or while on a vacation at home, the disease might be treated differently in each circumstance, but the basic principles of care would be the same. Similarly, although no two cases of hypothermia are alike, the principles of management are. Therapeutic success comes from understanding the principles of care and adapting them to the situation.

MILD VS PROFOUND HYPOTHERMIA

Patients with mild hypothermia must be distinguished from those with profound hypothermia. These two distinct groups have entirely different problems and mortality and therefore must be managed differently. Treating a patient with mild hypothermia as if he had profound hypothermia causes unnecessary inconvenience, expense, and discomfort, and may jeopardize other victims if resources are limited. Treating profound hypothermia as mild hypothermia endangers the victim's life.

Acute immersion hypothermia and chronic exposure hypothermia should be treated the same way. The environment in which each type of hypothermia occurs and the problems which may be encountered are different, but the principles of care are identical.

MILD HYPOTHERMIA (CORE TEMPERATURE ABOVE 90° F OR 32° C)

Mild hypothermia victims only need to be protected from further cooling and may be rewarmed by any convenient means. If placed in a warm environment, they will rewarm by themselves with no complications. Preventing further cooling requires enough understanding of the mechanisms by which heat is produced and heat is lost to take effective measures. (See Chapter One, "Control of Body Temperature," and Chapter Two, "Avoiding Hypothermia.")

Of particular concern is the person removed from cold water who can continue to cool rapidly unless further evaporative heat loss is prevented. Ideally, wet clothing should be replaced with dry clothing. If no dry clothing is available, the wet clothing should be wrung out to remove as much water as possible and put back on, if it has any insulating value. If the wet clothing must be left on, evaporative heat loss should be minimized by covering the individual with some impervious material, such as a raincoat or plastic sheets or bags

Warm liquids may be given by mouth, even though they have virtually no warming effect on core temperature. The number of calories in a cup or two of a warm beverage is quite small, but they can make a person feel warmer and more comfortable. When swallowed, the liquid warms the blood going to the brain, where the "thermostat" is located. The thermostat interprets this warm blood as a sensation of being too warm and responds with messages to the body to lose heat by sending more blood to the skin. The dilatation of blood vessels in the skin produces the warm feeling. The increased blood flow to the skin could increase heat loss and divert blood needed for more vital organs. However, the heat loss would be minimal if measures to reduce it have been taken, and the benefits from having the individual feel better are more significant. A safe guideline is that any mildly hypothermic patient capable of easily drinking warm liquids benefits from them. Alcohol produces a similar warm sensation, but its other effects are so deleterious that it should not be given to hypothermia victims.

A person with mild hypothermia can rewarm himself if heat loss is stopped, but external heat may be added safely by any means available. Heat sources such as hot water bottles, heating pads, or warm stones rewarm the body core most effectively when applied to the areas of least insulation, primarily the inguinal areas (where the thighs meet the trunk), sides of the chest, and head and neck. A second person in a sleeping bag can provide heat for gentle rewarming but not as effectively as other means. Submersion in hot water or a hot shower is safe with mild hypothermia but should be used only with absolute certainty that profound hypothermia is not present.

PROFOUND HYPOTHERMIA (CORE TEMPERATURE BELOW 90°F OR 32° C)

The mortality from hypothermia so profound that the victim is unconscious varies from fifty to eighty percent, even when patients have been brought alive into hospital emergency rooms. This condition is a life threatening, true medical emergency which must be treated as such. When death occurs during treatment, it is invariably from ventricular fibrillation, an abnormal heart rhythm that prevents the heart from pumping blood. This abnormal rhythm almost never reverts to normal spontaneously, and usually can not be stopped, even with the best treatment available, in severely hypothermic patients.

The fundamental principle of care for patients with profound hypothermia consists of avoiding ventricular fibrillation while the victims slowly rewarm.

Listed below are some of the events known to have triggered ventricular fibrillation in victims of profound hypothermia:

Table 4. Events Known to Trigger Ventricular Fibrillation
in Patients with Profound Hypothermia

1. Endotracheal intubation
2. Rapid assisted positive pressure ventilation (mouth to mouth resuscitation)
3. Alkalosis caused by excessive intravenous sodium bicarbonate
4. Precordial thump
5. Inserting a large bore needle into central veins
6. Physical exertion
7. Rough handling while lifting or transporting
8. Inserting endocardial catheters or pacing wires
9. Rapid external rewarming
10. Cardiac stimulating medications, including isoproterenol and epinephrine

Physical Exertion

Sudden death has been observed when victims of profound hypothermia lie still—or float—for prolonged periods and then physically exert themselves. This complication has been encountered most commonly in victims of cold water immersion who have started swimming to reach a rescue boat or have tried to pull themselves into the boat.

When the patient with profound hypothermia is lying or floating still, the blood circulation to the extremities is greatly reduced. Blood already in the extremities remains there and becomes colder and more metabolically bankrupt, with a high acid and potassium content and low oxygen. When the arms or legs are used, after being immobile for so long, the muscular action pumps the blood back to the heart. This organ, already compromised by the cold, is suddenly hit by even colder blood containing the irritating products of anaerobic metabolism. Ventricular fibrillation is the common result.

To avoid this lethal complication, the victim of profound hypothermia must never exert himself. He must not walk, climb, swim, or even move when lifted. If the victim is in cold water, he must not try to climb into the boat, but should allow himself to be carefully and gently lifted from the water. Similarly, the rescuers should avoid pumping venous blood into the central circulation by minimizing their manipulation of the victim's extremities. Some authorities have recommended that wet trousers not be removed for this reason.

Gentle Handling

Triggering ventricular fibrillation by physically jarring the heart of persons in profound hypothermia has been clearly demonstrated in animal experiments and in humans during induced hypothermia (mostly to allow interruption of the circulation during heart surgery). This catastrophe is well exemplified by the victim who is alive when placed in a rescue sled but dead fifteen minutes later, after a bumpy ride down the mountain, or by the victim who dies while being roughly lifted from a stretcher onto an examining table in the hospital emergency room. Patients in profound hypothermia must be handled as carefully and as gently as patients with fractures of the cervical spine. Such gentle handling may be difficult during a water or mountain rescue, but the rescuer really has no choice. The rescue will be futile if not carried out gently. Furthermore, a victim who has been cold for some time suffers little adverse effect from the few additional minutes required to provide careful, gentle handling.

Rewarming in the Field

Most persons in the United States with extensive experience treating semiconscious or unconscious hypothermia patients think victims of profound hypothermia should not be rewarmed outside of a hospital unless absolutely no alternative exists. Rapid rewarming may lead to "rewarming shock" and ventricular fibrillation. Rewarming shock, which is not completely understood, occurs when a victim of profound hypothermia who is also severely dehydrated — a common combination — is immersed in warm water. The blood vessels in the extremities, which have previously been constricted, dilate in response to the warmth. The blood in the body core, already reduced in volume by dehydration, is shunted to the periphery, resulting in a severe fall in blood pressure and shock. The cold, metabolically imbalanced blood in the arms and legs is returned to the heart, causing a further drop in the core temperature and sometimes initiating ventricular fibrillation. Even though the mechanisms of rewarming shock, temperature "after drop," and ventricular fibrillation are not fully understood, their occurrence with rapid external rewarming has been observed too many times to be questioned.

For these reasons, no attempt should be made to rapidly rewarm an unconscious profoundly hypothermic individual outside of a hospital. Under most circumstances no rewarming at all should be attempted.

If the victim is stable, gets no colder, and no one tampers with him, he can remain safely in his "metabolic icebox" for hours or even days. If gentle transportation to a hospital can be obtained within a few hours, the safest approach is to NOT add external heat. If transfer to a hospital is totally impossible, the very gentle application of heat—at first to the trunk alone – may succeed in raising body temperature.

In certain circumstances, particularly after removal from cold water, the core temperature may continue to drop as the result of the influx of cold blood from the extremities. In such situations an argument can be made for the gentle application of heat to the trunk.

Heated, Humidified Air or Oxygen

Treatment of hypothermia victims in the field or in hospital emergency rooms with heated, humidified air or oxygen has received much attention in recent years because it appears to provide a simple, easily portable means for introducing heat directly into the core—the lungs and then the heart—of a hypothermia victim. Although this technique can be useful, it has severe limitations which must be kept in mind before electing to administer such therapy.

The amount of heat carried by the oxygen or the air in such systems is insignificant because almost all of the heat is transmitted by the water used to humidify the air. Most of this heat is released when the water condenses in the lungs or the respiratory passages. If not humidified, heated air or oxygen might actually have an overall cooling effect caused by the evaporation of air to humidify the gases as they pass through the major air passages.

Such systems are capable of transmitting only a very small amount of heat, largely because the specific heat of gases is so small. At a respiratory rate of ten liters per minute, the maximum heat input has been estimated at 10 kilocalories per hour. For comparison, an adult male of average size with a normal body temperature while sitting quietly produces 70 to 100 kilocalories per hour—seven to ten times as much heat—by basal metabolism alone. A hypothermic individual produces significantly less heat this way.

Even these figures tend to exaggerate the amount of heat transferred. Normal respiratory volume is approximately 7.5 liters per minute and only two-thirds of that reaches the lungs where heat can be effectively transferred. The other one-third fills the nose, throat, trachea, and bronchi. Furthermore, profoundly hypothermic individuals breathe slower and shallower than normal.

For heated humidified gases to be most effective, they should be administered through an endotracheal tube. However, tracheal intubation is hazardous because it may cause ventricular fibrillation, although the significance of this hazard is debated. Furthermore, if the victim's breathing is controlled with a bag attached to the system, overventilation can occur, producing respiratory alkalosis and increasing the risk of ventricular fibrillation.

Another problem associated with the administration of heated, humidified gases is the possibility that rescuers could be lulled into a false sense that they are doing much more for the victim than they really are, thereby failing to aggressively pursue efforts to protect him from the cold and get him evacuated. Almost any cold exposure would cause heat loss far greater than the few calories a heated, humidified gas system could add.

In spite of these limitations, such systems are not without value. Heat loss from the respiratory tract can be as high as 13 kilocalories per hour. A heated gas system can prevent such losses as well as add an additional 10 kilocalories per hour—a total swing of 23 kilocalories per hour. A calorie saved is a calorie that does not have to be replaced later.

A number of devices to heat oxygen or air are suitable for field use and commercially available. However, the most valuable place for such devices may be in hospital emergency rooms for use after heat loss to the environment has been stopped or for those situations in which evacuation is impossible.

Mouth-to mouth assisted ventilation has been suggested as a means of adding heat to the core. The amount of heat added would be similar to that provided by heated, humidified gases – about nine kilocalories per hour. In a cold environment respiratory heat losses of the same magnitude would be prevented. However, the dangers of overventilation are real.

Table 5. Summary of Basic Management for
Profound Hypothermia Outside of a Hospital

1. No physical exertion
2. Gentle handling
3. No rapid rewarming (immersion in hot water)

ADVANCED LIFE SUPPORT

Because well staffed rescue groups include emergency medical personnel or physicians who are capable of administering advanced life support, a review of the basic principles of advanced support for victims of profound hypothermia seems merited.

Intravenous Therapy

Intravenous administration of fluids to expand the circulation is a valuable aspect of advanced life support. Most hypothermia victims are dehydrated and have a reduced circulating blood volume. (See Chapter Three, "Reponses to Cooling.") As the victim warms and the blood vessels in the periphery dilate, blood filling those vessels becomes unavailable to the vital organs of the core – the heart, lungs, and brain – thereby further impairing the effectiveness of the blood circulation.

Rapidly expanding the blood volume by infusing intravenous fluids could elevate blood pressure, increasing blood flow through the coronary arteries and oxygen delivery to the heart muscle. Improvement of blood circulation to the heart would decrease the risk of rewarming shock and fatal ventricular fibrillation. However, the peripheral blood vessels of severely hypothermic persons are commonly so constricted that inserting an intravenous line is very difficult and may be impossible.

Large-bore needles introduced into the large central veins may trigger ventricular fibrillation, so large peripheral veins should be used. Any crystalloid solution, such as lactated Ringers', or saline, is suitable. The fluid should not be colder than body temperature; warming the fluid to 104°F (40° C) is ideal because some warmth is provided in addition to the fluid itself. Initially, 300 cc should be given very rapidly, preferably before the patient is moved. The remaining 700 cc or so can be administered in twenty to thirty minutes. If more fluids are available, they must be administered more slowly, unless the victim is very large or unusually dehydrated.

Cardiac Resuscitation

Profoundly hypothermic individuals with no effective cardiac function – ventricular fibrillation or asystole (no heart beat at all) – or blood circulation can survive for only about sixty to ninety minutes without sustaining significant neurologic damage. CPR is required when evacuation requires more than a few minutes.

Individuals with a detectable heart beat should not receive CPR because ventricular fibrillation would usually result. At least one full minute – preferably three – should be spent trying to detect a carotid pulse before assuming a hypothermia victim has no effective cardiac activity. Portable EKG monitors are often required for detecting cardiac activity in victims of severe hypothermia and whenever possible should be carried by rescue groups. In wilderness situations EKG's can determine that normal cardiac electrical activity is present, even though they cannot reliably distinguish between asystole, ventricular fibrillation, or baseline artifacts.

If CPR is needed, it should be administered according to the standards established by the American Heart Association. It should be initiated in the field only by an experienced team that can also provide advanced life support. CPR should not be started until the team and the victim are in a safe, protected environment.

If the individual is fibrillating, successful electrical defibrillation is unlikely until the body has been rewarmed to a temperature of 90° to 92° F (32° to 33° C). If an initial countershock is unsuccessful, repeated shocks may be harmful and should be avoided until the victim has been rewarmed.

CPR clearly should be instituted following a witnessed cardiac arrest, particularly when transport to a hospital is expected to require more than a few minutes. CPR should probably be administered to individuals with unwitnessed cardiac arrest who appear resuscitatable, but each situation is so unique that more definitive recommendations are not possible.

CPR should not be instituted for severe hypothermia victims who can be transported to a hospital in minutes, particularly when the need for stretcher evacuation or similar circumstances prevents the administration of effective CPR. A hostile environment may require that CPR be postponed or abandoned entirely.

Preferably, profound hypothermia victims with no cardiac function should be evacuated to a hospital with a cardiac surgery service. The heart-lung machine (extracorporeal bypass) used for such surgery can rewarm the victim more rapidly than other techniques and can allow cardiac function to be restored before irrecoverable neurologic damage has occurred.

Successful resuscitation of profound hypothermia victims has been achieved in amazing circumstances. In a safe environment, resuscitative efforts should not be abandoned until hope is unequivocally lost – usually only after the victim has been rewarmed.

Clearly, hypothermia should be avoided, not treated.

Drugs

Most drugs are inactive or ineffective at profoundly hypothermic body temperatures. Bicarbonate is of little help in correcting the metabolic acidosis ubiquitous in profound hypothermia; an excess can predispose the victim to ventricular fibrillation. Other drugs often used following cardiac arrest in normothermic persons, such as atropine, isoproterenol, and epinephrine, can induce ventricular fibrillation in hypothermic individuals. Drugs are metabolized more slowly during hypothermia, which can lead to accumulations that are toxic when normal temperature is restored.

A SCENARIO

A party of three elk hunters has been comfortably camped deep in the wilderness. The ground is covered with snow, and the temperature is below freezing. In the morning they leave in different directions, planning to rendezvous at camp for lunch. Only two return. After a respectable wait they follow the third's tracks to their end at a log crossing a steam of moderate size. After following downstream for thirty minutes, the hunters find their companion on a small rocky beach. He is soaking wet with one foot still in the water. His hat is gone and his jacket is open. He is obviously dazed and confused but responds slightly to their presence. He is lying face down and tries to move when they approach.

Diagnosis

Profound hypothermia must be suspected at once in view of the victim's situation, his wet clothing, the cold environment, and the elapsed time since he was last seen. His failure to remove himself completely from the water, to keep his jacket zipped or otherwise protect himself from the cold, as well as his confused behavior, further suggest the diagnosis.

Treatment

1. The victim must not be allowed to move – not to stand up, sit up, or even roll over.
2. The victim must be examined to see if he is having difficulty breathing and to check for injuries such as gunshot wounds or fractures, particularly a fractured neck. A clear airway should be established.
3. The victim should gently be removed from the water.
4. Further heat loss must be prevented:
   a. Wet clothing should be removed and gently replaced with whatever dry clothing can be donated. Items which can not be replaced should be wrung out and put back on, particularly woolen clothing. Down clothing should be avoided. The head, neck, and trunk must be well covered.
   b. The victim should be covered with any available ground cloths, raincoats, or blankets.
   c. Boots or constricting garments must be loosened to prevent frostbite.
   d. Insulation from the ground should be provided with boughs, leaves, grass, or any available material.
   e. A fire should be built, if possible, using a backdrop to reflect more heat.
   f. The four mechanisms of heat loss – convection, conduction, radiation, and evaporation – should be reviewed to ensure no avenues of heat escape have been overlooked.
5. Plans for a definitive camp should be made:
   a. If possible, the original camp can be moved to the victim.
   b. If the camp can not be moved, a makeshift stretcher should be constructed to transport the patient to the camp. He should not be carried on a rescuer's back.
   c. While one person sets up camp or builds a stretcher, the other should stay with the victim to prevent activity and perhaps provide some body warmth. When applying body-to-body warmth, as

little clothing should be between the two as possible.

6. The victim should be placed inside a shelter – a tent will do if nothing better is available, but snow caves or similar shelters are warmer:

   a. The four mechanisms of heat loss should again be reviewed to ensure that no method of prevention has been overlooked.

   b. The shelter should be warmed with a stove or by rocks that have been brought in after being heated outside.

   c. Body-to-body contact should be used to warm the victim, if necessary.

   d. If the victim is not rewarming after two hours and definitive rescue is distant, heat should be gently applied to the trunk with heated stones or hot water containers. (The heated objects must not burn the victim.)

7. Plans for a definitive rescue should be made.

ADDITIONAL READING

Harnett RM, Pruitt JR, Sias FR: A review of the literature concerning resuscitation from hypothermia: Part I – the problem and general approaches. *Aviat Space Environ Med* 1983;54:425-434.

Harnett RM, Pruitt JR, Sias FR: A review of the literature concerning resuscitation form hypothermia: Part II – selected rewarming protocols. *Aviat Space Environ Med* 1983;54:487-495.

CHAPTER SIX

Immersion Hypothermia

JOHN S. HAYWARD, PH.D.

Some of the most enjoyable outdoor recreational activities—sailing and windsurfing, fishing, river running, scuba and skin diving, and power boating—take place on lakes, rivers, and oceans. The pleasure of water related activities should not be spoiled by water's lethal potential for drowning and hypothermia. Personal flotation devices (PFDs) can largely eliminate the risk of drowning, but the problem of immersion hypothermia is more difficult and deserves thoughtful consideration by everyone at risk of accidental immersion in cold water.

The threat of hypothermia during immersion derives from two specific characteristics of water: the great speed with which it can conduct heat (thermal conductivity), and the large amount of heat required to raise its temperature (specific heat). These two properties, combined with water's ability to penetrate clothing and make excellent thermal contact with the body surface, produce high rates of heat loss from the body if the water is cold. In an average person these high rates of heat loss easily exceed the capacity for sustained heat production in water as slightly cold as the low 70s F (low 20s C). Such heat loss leads to a rapid temperature decline, first in the peripheral tissues and subsequently in the core.

Many experimental studies of immersion hypothermia have been made during the last two to three decades. The information gained from these studies, together with analyses of accidental immersions in cold water, has provided a reasonably good understanding of this topic and permits some recommendations for avoiding or dealing with such accidents.

Cold water can kill in several ways. These can be discussed as "short term" and "long term immersion."

SHORT TERM COLD WATER IMMERSION

Heart Dysfunction

When the body is suddenly immersed in cold water, the shock from the immediate, drastic cooling of the skin can elicit several responses from the circulatory and respiratory systems. The blood pressure can rise rapidly due to a simultaneous constriction of the peripheral blood vessels and an increase in heart rate induced by the victim's alarm. Persons with weak hearts and circulatory systems, such as many elderly individuals, may develop lethal cardiac functional abnormalities at this time. Even young, healthy persons occasionally can develop abnormalities of the heart beat (arrhythmias), which may cause sudden death.

Breathing Abnormalities

Another initial response to cold water immersion is hyperventilation, an increase in the rate and depth of breathing. The first few seconds of immersion are characterized by huge, involuntary gasps. These are followed by a minute or more of rapid, deep breaths, which increase breathing volume to about five times that of normal resting levels. The immersion victim feels that he can not "catch his breath." The likelihood for unintentionally aspirating water and drowning is greatly increased, particularly if the person plunges underwater or if the water is turbulent and high waves are present.

A further complication of hyperventilation is alkalosis. The increased ventilation causes larger quantities of carbon dioxide to be lost through the lungs, significantly reducing the amount of carbon dioxide in the blood, and increasing in the blood pH. If severe, these changes can reduce the flow of blood to the brain, resulting in dizziness or fainting and an increased probability of drowning.

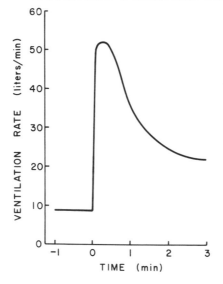

Figure 1. Typical hyperventilation response upon sudden immersion in cold water.

Another way cold water increases the likelihood of death during the early phase of accidental immersion is by limiting the victim's ability to hold his breath. The breath holding capacity of an average individual in water colder than 60° F (15° C) is in the range of fifteen to twenty-five seconds, approximately one-third of normal. If a person were submerged below the surface after accidental immersion, such as capsizing in a turbulent river or being trapped in a sinking vessel, the reduced time which he could hold his breath would definitely increase his risk of drowning.

Muscle Dysfunction

As part of the early response to immersion in cold water, the blood vessels in the skin and skeletal muscles constrict strongly. This constriction leads to the establishment of an outer "shell" that cools more quickly than the core and thereby provides an important means of reducing further heat loss. However, such "tissue insulation" can hasten death in certain circumstances. Cooling of the muscles and the nerves supplying them results in slower, weaker, poorly coordinated movements. The ability to swim or tread water is greatly impaired.

Even good swimmers drown more quickly unless they are wearing PFDs or holding on to floating objects. Muscular dysfunction increases with the coldness of the water. Inability to continue swimming commonly occurs within ten to fifteen minutes after immersion in water colder than 50° F (10° C).

Importantly, this slowing and weakening of muscular function affects more than just the ability to swim. A victim immersed more than ten minutes in cold water (five minutes in icy water) is less able to climb onto a floating object or to catch and put on a PFD, rescue sling, or other rescue device which may be thrown to him. In such cases the rescuer must be prepared to enter the water with the victim to aid in his recovery.

Precautions

Death in the early phases of immersion clearly does not result from core hypothermia. With the exception of cardiac arrhythmias, such deaths are drownings caused by cold induced breathing irregularities or muscular abnormalities.

Most persons immersed in cold water do not die immediately, but the possibility is great enough to warrant taking some precautions. If possible, the water should be entered gradually, with the head well clear of waves or turbulence. No one should dive into cold water, even if it is deep. Breathing should be consciously controlled as much as possible during entry and for the subsequent minute or two until the feeling of being unable to "catch one's breath" has disappeared. The more clothing and insulation being worn, the less the hyperventilatory response. Of course, a PFD is a vital precaution.

LONG TERM COLD WATER IMMERSION

Very few victims of accidental immersion in cold water who have some means of flotation die from short term problems. Most face a much slower death. After ten to fifteen minutes of immersion, shivering becomes conspicuous and continuous. The victim feels miserable and appreciates the dilemma of cold water immersion in a way impossible to achieve by reading about it. Persons rescued at this stage often make statements such as, "I couldn't have lasted much longer." Though inaccurate, such assessments do reflect how badly the victims feel and how terrible they appear to observers. They also may contribute to the false impression that death from hypothermia can occur after only minutes in cold water. Actually, fifteen to twenty minutes must elapse before the body core begins to cool consistently.

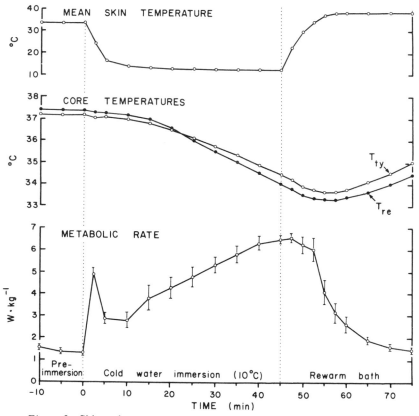

Figure 2. Skin and core temperatures (T_{ty} = tympanic; T_{re} = rectal) and metabolic rates of seminude, nonexercising adult humans immersed in cold water and subsequently rewarmed in warm water. Metabolic rate increases are mostly the result of shivering. Core temperatures begin to decline only after about fifteen minutes of immersion. During rewarming, metabolic rates (and the sensation of coldness) decline rapidly after the skin temperature is raised to normal, even though core temperatures are at their lowest point.

Experimental Immersion Hypothermia

The average responses of ten nonexercising, seminude, male subjects immersed in 50° F (10° C) water and rewarmed in a bath are presented in Figure 2. Within five to ten minutes, their skin temperatures had dropped nearly to that of the water. Their metabolic rates (heat production) had risen dramatically in response to their initial shock and then settled to a level about two times higher than before immersion. After fifteen to twenty minutes, their core temperatures (measured at rectal and tympanic sites) began to fall consistently. Shivering and metabolic rates increased in proportion to the core cooling. When their core temperatures had reached 93° to 95° F (34° to 35° C), maximum levels of shivering occurred and heat production was four to five times greater than before immersion. However, all of the heat produced by shivering failed to halt the decline of core temperature into hypothermia. The body's ability to produce extra heat by shivering may be sufficient to temporarily offset heat losses in still, cold air, but not in cold water.

Physiologic changes that accompanied cooling (but which are not presented in Figure 2) included increases in the heart rates to as much as 150 per minute, in blood concentrations of noradrenaline, and in urine volumes to about three times normal (cold diuresis). Changes in intellectual function, such as a lessened ability to maintain a logical sequence of ideas, were also present in mildly hypothermic subjects. This may account for the strange and inappropriate behavior often seen in hypothermia victims.

During the rewarming phase of the studies, shivering ceased when the skin temperature returned to normal, even though the core temperature was continuing to fall (afterdrop). Ten to fifteen minutes after entering the warm bath, the subjects felt good, even though their core temperatures were then at their lowest, demonstrating that the sensation of cold is only skin deep. The relevance of this finding is considered in a later discussion of differences between the way an immersion victim feels and the way he cools.

Cooling and Survival Time

After fifteen to twenty minutes, a graph of the core temperatures of persons immersed in cold water and unprotected by special survival clothing forms a fairly straight line (Figure 2). Other evidence indicates that cooling continues in a similar linear fashion down to levels of profound hypothermia. Accordingly, various investigators have been able to determine cooling rates of the body in water of different temperatures and have used these rates to predict survival times. Average rectal cooling rates at different water temperatures are listed in Table 6.

Table 6. Average Core Cooling Rates for Nonexercising,
Lightly Clothed Adults During Immersion in
Cold Water of Different Temperatures

Water Temperature		Cooling Rate
(°F)	(°C)	(°C/hour)
68	20	0.5
59	15	1.5
50	10	2.5
41	5	4.0
32	0	6.0

To predict survival times from such cooling data requires the selection of an endpoint, a core temperature at which death is probable, and an acceptable definition of death based on cessation of respiratory and cardiac function. (Victims of profound hypothermia have been resuscitated even though these functions were absent, thanks to the protective effect of hypothermia. See Chapter Five, "Treatment of Hypothermia.") A reasonable choice for victims of water immersion is 86° F (30° C) because at this temperature victims are usually semiconscious and likely to drown. Additionally, below this temperature the probability of heart irregularities is increased.

Figure 3 is a graph that predicts average survival time to a core temperature of 86° F (30° C) at different water temperatures. It includes the distribution of predicted survival times for victims who cool faster or slower than the average (see below). The data were derived from persons who were holding still while wearing a standard lifejacket and light clothing. For example, the estimated survival time in 50° F (10° C) water is about two and one-half to three hours for the average person. Recent experimental findings have

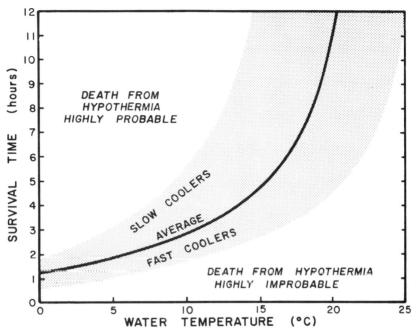

Figure 3. Predicted survival times for lightly clothed, nonexercising humans in cold water. The grey zone includes approximately ninety-five percent of the variation expected for adult and teenage humans.

confirmed a potential average survival time for persons who hold still while immersed in ice water (32° F or 0° C) of just over an hour. Only when the water temperature is above 60° F (15° C) is the average, potential survival time long enough for search and rescue operations to have a high probability of success. Since much recreational and commercial boating is done in water below this temperature, particularly in the spring and fall, the risk of hypothermic death is considerable. As a rule of thumb, if no one is swimming at the beaches, a significant potential for hypothermia is present.

Individual Variation in Cooling Rate

Figure 3 also illustrates the rather large individual differences in cooling rates and predicted survival times. Differences in body build have a great effect on cooling rate, and body fat is the major determinant of that rate in humans. Fat people have long been known to cool more slowly than lean ones. (The protection of subcutaneous fat possibly could be called the "blubber effect" in recognition of the way warm blooded, aquatic mammals such as seals or whales use such insulation to prevent core hypothermia.)

For most aspects of human health, excess fat is a liability; in cold water it is an asset! Fat has a relatively low blood flow and therefore is able to provide a shell of insulation for the body core. Subcutaneous fat is considered an important prerequisite for long distance swimmers, particularly in relatively cold water such as the English Channel, and is largely responsible for the cold water exploits of the famous Korean women divers. Studies in Britain and France have produced the generalization that doubling the skinfold thickness (a common measure of subcutaneous fat) halves the cooling rate. Estimated survival time in water of 50° F (10° C) would be only one and one-half hours for a very lean person with an average skinfold thickness of 5 mm, but would be six hours for a fat person with an average skinfold thickness of 20 mm.

Body size, as distinct from fatness, also influences the cooling rate in cold water. Because the ratio of surface area to volume increases as the size of a body decreases, large individuals cool more slowly than small ones, even if both have the same thickness of subcutaneous fat. Children cool most rapidly because they have small bodies, usually with relatively little fat. Women commonly have more fat under their skin than men, which would tend to enable them to last longer in cold water. However, because this advantage is offset by their significantly smaller average body size, they often cool at nearly the same rate as men. These body variables can not be readily changed and therefore can not be considered appropriate "strategies" for dealing with accidental immersion in cold water.

Influence of Alcohol

Consumption of alcoholic beverages is frequently a component of many aquatic activities, such as recreational boating or fishing. Blood alcohol concentrations above the legally defined level of impairment, which ranges from 0.05 to 0.10 gm of alcohol per 100 ml of blood, are not at all uncommon. Such blood alcohol concentrations certainly increase the chances of accidentally entering the water and probably reduce the victim's ability to get back out by swimming or other means. However, moderate amounts of alcohol do not appear to increase the speed with which hypothermia develops.

Alcohol has been known for some time to dilate peripheral blood vessels and slightly lower the body temperature of humans in normal environments (no cold stress). However, recent studies have found that alcohol concentrations below 0.10 g/100 ml do not significantly affect the rate of cooling in cold water or in cold air. Apparently, the strong stimulus of a cold skin overwhelms the mild anesthetic effect of the alcohol so that peripheral blood vessel constriction and muscular shivering take place in an almost normal manner. Undoubtedly, a greater degree of intoxication, perhaps to the point of stupor, would impair these mechanisms and result in a faster cooling rate. As with so many phenomena, the effects are dose dependent.

In summary, *the basic, involuntary thermoregulatory responses of the human body are inadequate for maintaining normal body temperature during immersion in cold water.*

COLD WATER SAFETY

When faced with physiologic limitations, humans intellectually devise methods for overcoming those limitations. Technological devices and modified behavior can extend man's limited ability to survive the hypothermia resulting from cold water immersion. For deliberate immersion, such as scuba diving, excellent devices—wet suits and dry suits—have been developed. Within recent years, as the significance of accidental cold water immersion has been more widely recognized, behavioral and technologic methods for reducing the severity of this hazard also have been developed.

Swimming

The heat produced by physical activity is known to play a major role in maintaining body temperature in cold air. Is the same true for accidental cold water immersion? Can a strong swimmer power his way out of trouble through muscular activities that produce heat faster than shivering? The answer is No!—absolutely and unequivocally!

In cold water physical activity increases heat loss more than it increases heat production. Activities such as swimming accelerate the core cooling rate by thirty-five to fifty percent, particularly in water colder than 60° F (15° C). Physical activity forces water through clothing and around the body, thereby accelerating heat loss by convection. More importantly, physical activity stimulates blood circulation to the body's periphery, particularly the muscles of the arms and legs, in the process greatly reducing its primary defense mechanism against cold water—an outer shell of cold tissue which acts as insulation for the core. Figure 4 illustrates this point with infrared photographs which show the relative surface temperatures of the upper body. Dark regions are colder; light regions are warmer. The thermograms illustrate the differences in surface temperature, and consequent heat loss, (a) prior to immersion, (b) after immersion while holding still, and (c) after immersion while swimming.

Prior to immersion, the body surface has a fairly uniform temperature, warmest in the armpits. When the subject holds still after immersion, most of the body surface is cold, indicating the presence of a cool outer shell of tissue (skin and subcutaneous tissue). The areas of highest heat loss are along the sides of the chest and in the inguinal areas, where the body wall is thin, or large blood vessels are near the surface. When the subject swims after immersion, the body surface is warmer and heat loss is greater. The skin may even feel slightly warmer, giving an erroneous impression that swimming in this situation is beneficial. Clearly the sensation of warmth is misleading, because heat is being lost and the body core is cooling.

The advice to avoid physical activity in cold water must be modified, of course, to allow swimming to a nearby rescue vessel, or even to shore if a PFD is available (swimming in cold water without a PFD is suicidal) and the shore is close enough. What is close enough? The distance depends upon water temperature, wave action and water currents, swimming ability, body build, and the clothing worn. The only data available suggest that the average person is unlikely to be able to swim more than a kilometer (about six-tenths of

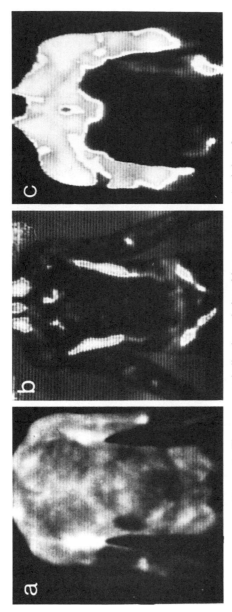

Figure 4. Thermograms indicating relative skin temperatures (and therefore relative heat loss): (a) before immersion in 45.5°F (7.5°C) water, (b) after holding still in the water for fifteen minutes, and (c) after swimming for fifteen minutes. Lighter areas are warmer.

a mile) in 50° F (10° C) water. At a distance from shore of one-half mile or more, the threat of hypothermic death is more compelling because an individual accidentally immersed in cold water is dependent upon someone else for rescue.

Clearly, the way to slow body cooling in cold water is not through increased heat production by voluntary physical activity. Survival is dependent upon finding methods to reduce the loss of heat to the water.

Personal Flotation Devices

In the United States only a small percentage of boaters routinely wear PFDs. When sudden immersion occurs and no flotation is available, physical activity is necessary to avoid drowning. One such activity is treading water, in which the arms and legs move continuously in various patterns to keep the head out of the water. Test subjects treading water had an average cooling rate one-third faster than subjects holding still in a PFD.

In addition to cooling faster, most people tire rapidly while treading water. For this reason, the most effective survival swimming technique ("drownproofing") consists of floating restfully with the lungs full of air, and raising the head out of the water every ten to fifteen seconds to take another breath. With this procedure, even nonswimmers can avoid drowning for many hours in warm water. Unfortunately, in cold water this behavior results in a body cooling rate about eighty percent faster than that of individuals who hold still in a PFD. When drownproofing, not only is the person active, but he is immersing his head, another area of high heat loss, along with the rest of his body. Of the various survival techniques that might be used following immersion in cold water, drownproofing leads most rapidly to death from hypothermia. However, if drownproofing is the only way an immersion victim can avoid drowning, he clearly has no choice but to use that technique and hope that rescue arrives before severe hypothermia develops.

The inappropriateness of the best survival swimming technique for cold water survival should be a powerful incentive for boaters and others near cold water to always wear a PFD. Drownproofing is a highly valuable water safety technique, but its use should be restricted to warm water. (Ideally, drownproofing should never be needed at all.)

Strategies for Reducing the Cooling Rate

Reducing the amount of the body surface directly exposed to water decreases heat loss. Huddling by two or more persons in cold water can reduce the cooling rate by about one-third, particularly if chest contact is maximized. Similarly, an individual can reduce his cooling rate by twenty-five to thirty percent by adopting a body posture which minimizes the area of exposed body surface. This principle is far more important than any specific posture, but an example of this kind of positioning is the "Heat Escape Lessening Posture" (HELP) illustrated in Figure 5. This concept is not novel and is related to instinctive thermoregulatory behavior common to all warm blooded animals. The thermal benefit of strategies for reducing the exposed surface area may be relatively small but can result in an extra thirty to sixty minutes of survival, which may be critical for rescue. Knowledge of this principle also promotes a desirable survival psychology by providing something tangible and useful for the victims to do in a desperate situation.

H.E.L.P. (Heat Escape Lessening Posture)

Huddle

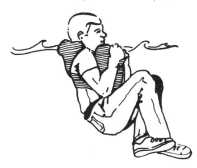
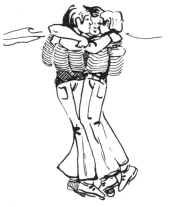

Figure 5. Methods for reducing the body surface area exposed to cold water.

The Effect of Clothing

Conventional clothing is designed to provide insulation in air, not water. When a person is immersed in cold water, protection by this clothing is greatly reduced. Due to its high heat capacity, even a small amount of water circulating through the clothing carries away a large amount of heat through convection. Additionally, the air spaces in the clothing are soon filled with water, which conducts heat away very rapidly. Attempts have been made to measure the insulation value of various types of standard clothing during water immersion. Heavy winter clothing increases the survival time above that expected with light clothing by about thirty to forty percent, which is clearly significant. Consequently, individuals who can foresee the need to enter cold water and who decide the shore is too distant for swimming should put on all of the clothing they can in the time available.

Removing shoes and clothing prior to entering the water is beneficial only for swimming. The clothing does increase the resistance to movement in water and greatly increases the effort required. However, rapid swimming is rarely a necessity in accidental cold water immersion. Additionally, clothes and most shoes that feel heavy in air when wet are not heavy in water and do not tend to "drag down" the wearer.

The only type of clothing material which provides effective thermal protection during immersion is that which traps air in such a manner that it can not be displaced by water. Only foams, such as the neoprene rubber of scuba divers' wet suits, or completely waterproof garments, such as divers' dry suits, offer such protection.

Cooling Rates in Different PFDs

A PFD should not be called a "life preserver" or a "life jacket" for cold water unless it can protect the wearer against hypothermia as well as drowning. A good PFD should be acceptable to and comfortable for the wearer, should have good flotation characteristics, including face up stability, and should be highly visible. To be considered a "life jacket," the PFD must reduce convective and conductive heat loss to the water. Most PFDs provide insignificant thermal protection because water can flow freely between them and the wearers. Vest PFDs that are made of foam and can be adjusted to fit snugly against the chest (usually with laces or straps at the sides and a front zipper) do provide some thermal protection in the water. A thick layer of closed cell foam closely applied to much of the chest can decrease the cooling rate by about thirty percent.

A further improvement in thermal protection is offered by flotation jackets, often called "float-coats." Flotation jackets that contain insulating foam and use special means to reduce water access to the body have been found to slow the rate of cooling in cold water by forty to fifty percent, which more than doubles the predicted survival time for a person with a noninsulating PFD. Wearing such jackets is much like wearing the top of a wet suit, except the garment's true character is disguised. A jacket attractive enough for general wear that also provides flotation and a measure of thermal protection in both cold air and water is of obvious value for boating in cool weather.

Cold Water Survival Suits

Survival or anti-exposure suits provide the most effective means for avoiding immersion hypothermia. These full body garments, used mostly for military or commercial activities (such as commercial fishing in cold water), are usually expensive and often uncomfortable and inconvenient to wear. The most thermally protective types keep the wearer dry and insulate against conductive heat loss with air that is trapped in closed cell foam or in heavy clothing worn beneath a waterproof garment. Models which are not waterproof rely upon closed cell foam for insulation, just as scuba divers' wet suits do. Some suits based on the wetsuit principle look like ordinary coveralls. Because they are easily donned, fairly comfortable to wear, moderately priced, and easily maintained, they are quite adaptable to recreational use, particularly for groups such as offshore sailors. These coverall suits can increase predicted survival time in cold water as much as four to five times that of an unprotected person.

Minimizing Submersion

Generally, the more of the body that is out of the water, the slower the core cooling rate. Therefore, accidental cold water immersion victims should make every effort to get out of the water onto a floating object, such as a log or their overturned boat. Even raising only the upper body from the water can greatly reduce cooling. Unfortunately, convenient floating objects are seldom available. New regulations for small boats, which require them to contain bouyant structures which make them float level when filled with water, should provide more immersion victims with a way to get out of the water. Badly needed is a small, inexpensive "miniraft" that could be carried as an accessory to a PFD and inflated when needed.

A person may feel just as cold, or even colder, when out of the water on a floating object as he would immersed, particularly if there is a wind. However, experimental studies and analyses of accidents have clearly documented a more rapid progress into core hypothermia when the victim is immersed in cold water. Again, the sensation of cold can be deceptive about core cooling. It is difficult to conceive of a realistic accident situation in which cold air, rain, and wind chill could match the heat loss caused by immersion in water at the same time and place.

Sublethal Effects of Immersion Hypothermia

Immersion hypothermia rarely produces any long term sublethal effects. If survivors are rewarmed effectively, they usually have no residual problems other than fatigue and some muscle soreness from shivering. A condition called "immersion foot" (or more commonly "trench foot") is a nonfreezing injury that occurs with prolonged, severe restriction of the blood flow to cold extremities, particularly the lower legs and feet. However, this disorder results from cold stress over a period of days, such as occurs in life rafts or lifeboats in cold regions. (See Chapter Eight, "Other Localized Cold Injuries.")

Acclimatization to Cold Water

Unfortunately, studies have shown no significant improvement in resistance to core cooling associated with repeated cold water im-

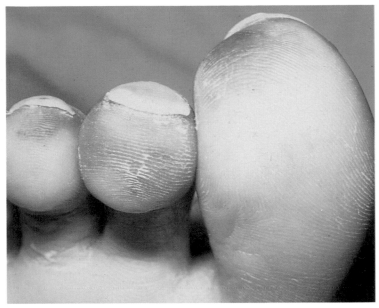

Figure A. Violaceous discoloration of the tips of the first three toes indicating mild frostbite. (This injury occurred in a young climber who was unaware that he had frostbite until he took off his boots in camp. No tissue loss resulted.) (Photograph courtesy Cameron C. Bangs, M.D.)

Figure B. Very early, mild frostbite of the toes and distal foot (blanched area) during rapid rewarming. Eventual tissue loss was limited to toe nails. (Photograph courtesy of Bruce C. Paton, M.D.)

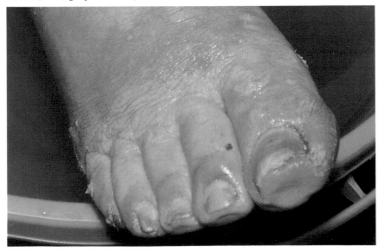

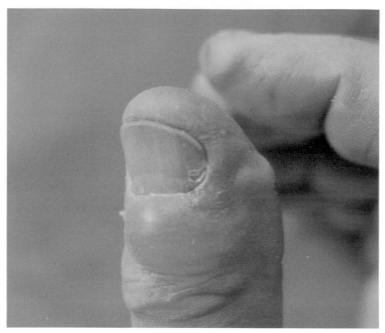

Figure C.

Figure D.

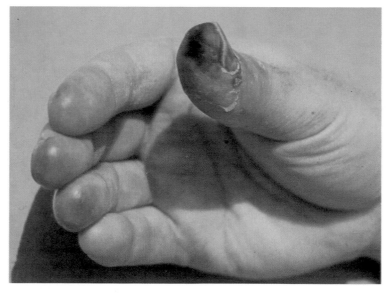

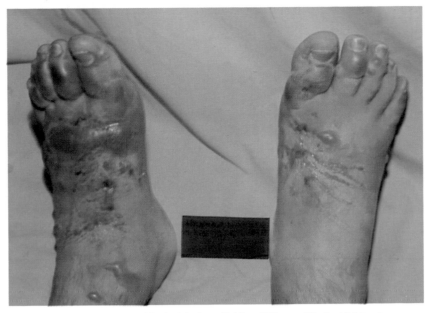

Figure E. Blisters filled with clear fluid and blisters filled with bloody fluid, neither extending to tips of toes, in relatively severe frostbite of the feet. (This injury resulted from sitting in the snow, meditating, with no protection for the feet but sneakers, for four hours.) (Photograph courtesy of Bruce C. Paton, M.D.)

Figure C. Bluish discoloration of the thumbnail and fingertips and a blister filled with clear fluid proximal to the nail (not extending to the tip of the thumb) in frostbite of moderate severity. (This injury occurred when a male climber took off one mitten during a severe blizzard only for long enough to urinate. The other hand was not injured. The photograph was taken one day later.)

Figure D. Blackened thumb tip and dark purple finger tips of the same hand one week later. (The site of the blister has a normal color and was less severely injured than the more distal tissues, which did not blister.)

(Photographs courtesy Cameron C. Bangs, M.D.)

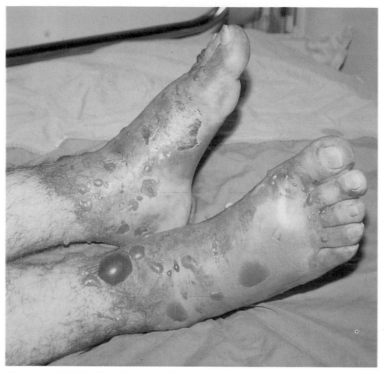

Figure F. Bluish discoloration, distal areas with no blisters, and more proximal areas covered by blisters, some filled with bloody fluid, on feet that have suffered severe frostbite. [This injury occurred in a man who spent twelve hours in a refrigerated railroad boxcar at 0° F (−18° C) wearing snugly laced, high top boots. His feet and ankles, which had their circulation impaired by the boots, were the only tissues that suffered cold injury.] Seven weeks after injury, the tissues not covered by blisters in this photograph are those that died, illustrating the difficulty of predicting the severity of tissue loss. Tissues covered by blisters containing bloody fluid usually die. (Photograph courtesy Cameron C. Bangs, M.D.)

mersion. No physiologic acclimatization that would reduce the rate of body cooling during an accident has been observed. Greater manual dexterity and reduced cold sensitivity have been observed, but these do not directly affect the rate at which core hypothermia develops. The only significant way to prepare for possible cold water immersion (other than wearing specialized clothing) is to increase body fat, which for most people is not an acceptable strategy.

Psychology of Cold Water Survival

Accounts of cold water immersion accidents often stress the importance of the victims' attitude or "psychology" for survival. The best "way of thinking" would permit the person to survive for the maximum time allowed by the physical factors controlling heat loss and heat production. A positive attitude can not prolong survival beyond the limits determined physically, but it is a vital element for achieving maximum survival and avoiding death from other causes. Victims who panic are incapable of survival behavior. Others without PFDs give up, let go of a floating object, and drown. Some fail to concentrate on keeping as much of the body out of the water as possible or maintaining a heat retaining posture. A strong "will to live," which is a component of a desirable psychological state, must dictate behavior that minimizes heat loss. An immersion victim who is not familiar with the body's responses to cold water immersion and the measures that can be taken to slow cooling is at a disadvantage for maintaining a strong and effective survival attitude when a real accident occurs.

ADDITIONAL READING

Cooper KE, Martin S, Riben P: Respiratory and other responses in subjects immersed in cold water. *J Appl Physiol* 1976; 40:903-910.

Hayward JS: The physiology of immersion hypothermia. In *The Nature and Treatment of Hypothermia*. Pozos R, Wittmers L, Jr: Ed. The University of Minnesota Press, Minneapolis, 1983.

Keatinge WR: *Survival in Cold Water*. Blackwell Scientific Publications, Oxford, 1969.

CHAPTER SEVEN

Frostbite

JAMES A. WILKERSON, M.D.

Frostbite is a localized cold injury characterized by freezing with ice crystal formation. This injury is almost always limited to the upper and lower extremities or to structures such as the ears or nose. The hands and feet do not contain large heat producing muscles and are a considerable distance from the major sites of heat generation. Furthermore, their blood supply is the first to be reduced when the body needs to conserve heat.

The toes are the most common site of frostbite, but the rest of the foot frequently is involved also. During outdoor activities in cold weather, the feet are in contact with ice or snow (through the shoes or boots) and are subjected to conductive heat loss as well as the radiant, convective, and evaporative heat loss that the rest of the body experiences. The fingers and hands are also common sites of frostbite and can suffer severe cold exposure if gloves or mittens are removed.

Minor frostbite injuries may also involve other tissues, such as the ears and tip of the nose. These structures are thin, easily chilled, and often exposed directly to wind. Although the resulting injuries are rarely severe—they are sometimes referred to as "frostnip"—they can be painful and disfiguring if tissue is actually lost. A common frostbite injury, at least before the manner in which it occurred became more widely known, was produced when a man's genitalia would come in contact with the metal zipper in the fly of his pants. This typically occurred in wearers of boxer undershorts who were preoccupied with whatever they were doing and did not notice the contact at the time it occurred.

Two other factors frequently contribute to the development of frostbite injuries of the hands and feet by reducing the blood supply to those tissues. The first is hypothermia. Although frostbite can occur without cooling of the entire body, hypothermia is usually present and causes constriction of the peripheral blood vessels in an effort to conserve heat for the body core. The second is obstruction of the blood supply to the extremities by constricting clothing. Boots laced too tightly are the most common offenders. Tight crampon straps are another. Plastic boots, which can not expand, have been commonly implicated in frostbite injuries, particularly when the boots have been lined with felt, which expands as it is wet by perspiration.

Contact with cold metal can produce very rapid and severe freezing of tissues. Minor injuries of this type have been experienced by most people through contact with metal ice cube trays, car door handles, or mailboxes during freezing temperatures. Deeper frostbite is possible from prolonged contact with larger objects, such as wrenches or jack handles, because metal is such an excellent conductor of heat.

However, much more severe injuries can be produced by organic liquids, such as gasoline or solvents, that have been left outdoors in below freezing weather. These fluids remain liquid at temperatures far below the freezing temperature of water and can absorb large quantities of heat. When they contact tissues, such supercooled liquids cause instantaneous freezing.

Frostbite only occurs at temperatures below freezing, but the actual temperature and time of exposure can vary considerably. Of 812 U.S. Army frostbite victims during the Korean conflict, eighty percent were injured at temperatures between 0° and 20° F (-18° to -7.5° C), and only ten percent were injured at lower temperatures. Sixty-seven percent of the victims had been immobilized by enemy fire, sleeping in a fox hole, or riding in a truck. Thirteen percent of the injuries occurred after less than seven hours of exposure, sixty-eight percent with seven to twelve hours, ten percent with thirteen to eighteen hours, and nine percent with longer than eighteen hours.

Predisposition to Frostbite

A number of studies carried out by military physicians have demonstrated an increased susceptibility to localized cold injury for certain groups of individuals. For example, blacks are three to six times more susceptible to frostbite than whites. Blacks do not increase their heat production as efficiently as whites, and they begin shivering at lower temperatures. Their fingers cool faster when immersed in cold water, reach a lower temperature before rewarming begins (hunting reaction), and do not rewarm as much as those of whites. The greater susceptibility of blacks to frostbite possibly is a result of long residence in tropical climates, where heat dissipation was more essential than heat conservation. Other evidence of a genetic predisposition to cold injury is an incidence of frostbite that is higher than expected in whites with type O blood and lower than expected in individuals with type A or type B blood.

Whether white or black, soldiers stationed in Alaska who were born in the southern part of the United States have an incidence of frostbite almost four times higher than soldiers born in the North. Moreover, individuals who had already spent one winter in Alaska had a lower incidence of frostbite than newcomers. Presumably, these differences result from greater experience in dealing with a cold environment, but the specific types of behavior that provide this protection have not been identified.

Lower military rank and educational level also are associated with a higher incidence of frostbite. Smokers have a higher incidence of frostbite than nonsmokers, presumably due to the vasoconstrictive effect of nicotine. Individuals who have previously suffered a cold injury have a greater risk of subsequent injury, but the reason is not clear because the second injury often involves a different part of the body.

Higher altitudes have been associated with a greater incidence of frostbite. Part of the increase is caused by the colder temperatures encountered at such elevations, but the hypoxia associated with altitude also diminishes resistance to cold injury. A reduction in cold induced vasodilatation (hunting reaction) at high altitudes has been demonstrated in individuals who were not native inhabitants of such elevations. The reduced vasodilatation persisted even after acclimatization. Additionally, the production of heat by metabolic processes other than muscular exercise (nonshivering thermogenesis) has been found to be reduced at high elevations.

Mechanisms of Tissue Injury

The tissue injury resulting from frostbite is produced in two ways. The most obvious is the actual freezing of the tissues. Although ice crystals form between the cells and grow by extracting water from them, the cells are physically disrupted by the ice crystals only to a limited extent. They are injured by the dehydration and osmotic and chemical imbalances resulting from extraction of water from within the cell, but permanent damage may be small. Under highly specific laboratory conditions frozen cells not only can survive for long periods of time but can grow in an appropriate cell culture medium after thawing. (Ice crystal formation within the cells, which would be much more destructive, requires much faster freezing than usually occurs with frostbite.)

The second mechanism of tissue injury by frostbite, which is much more significant, is obstruction of the blood supply to the tissues. The cells lining the capillaries and small veins (endothelial cells) in frostbitten tissues are damaged by the cold in such a manner that they allow the liquid part of the blood (the serum) to leak out into the tissues. Loss of this fluid diminishes the volume of the blood to such an extent that the rate of flow is greatly reduced. The blood cells no longer can remain suspended in the small volume of slowly moving serum and settle out or "sludge" within the vessels. Eventually the sludged blood clots, further obstructing the flow of blood, and circulation to the tissues ceases entirely.

Obstruction of the circulation by the sludging and subsequent clotting of blood plays a larger role in producing irreversible tissue damage than freezing. The changes produced in severely frostbitten tissues are identical to the damage caused by obstruction of the circulation by trauma or disease, such as arteriosclerosis (hardening of the arteries), in limbs that have not been exposed to cold. More recently, analyses of the fluid within the blisters that develop after frostbitten tissues are thawed have disclosed the presence of significant quantities of substances that promote clotting, such as prostaglandin F_{2a} and thromboxane B_2, which are released from damaged endothelial cells.

The circulation of blood to frostbitten extremities is usually severely impaired before frostbite occurs because the blood vessels are strongly constricted to conserve body heat. Indeed, such vasoconstriction can be so marked that circulation to the fingers or toes almost ceases. Nonetheless, the cold tends to protect the tissues from the effects of the diminished blood supply because the metabolism in the cells is so greatly reduced. In contrast, after thawing the cells are warm, metabolically active, and desperately in need of a good blood supply. An impaired blood supply at that time—which is the typical condition—would be far more damaging.

Prevention

In an environment in which the temperature is below freezing, frostbite can only be prevented by wearing protective clothing that prevents hypothermia of the entire body and protects the feet and hands.

Obstruction of the circulation must be avoided. Boots must not be laced too tightly; crampon straps must be loosened during rest periods; encircling, tightly fitting clothing must not be worn.

Cigarette smoking, or nicotine from any source, constricts the peripheral blood vessels and tends to aggravate local cold injuries. Alcohol tends to dilate blood vessels and might help prevent frostbite, but alcohol abuse is one of the most common elements predisposing to frostbite injuries because people do such stupid things under the influence of alcohol. (Exposure to severely cold conditions, such as immersion in cold water, overcomes the vasodilatation produced by moderate amounts of alcohol, and the blood vessels constrict.) Nicotine, particularly cigarettes, and alcohol should be avoided in environments cold enough to produce cold injuries.

Frostbite of the ears and nose can be avoided by keeping those areas covered and out of the wind, particularly while in a moving vehicle such as a snowmobile, or during fast skiing. Frostbite of the corneas of the eyes, a rare injury usually produced by exposure of the eyes to cold air while moving rapidly in similar circumstances, and treatable only by corneal transplantation, can be prevented by protective goggles.

DIAGNOSIS

The earliest symptom of frostbite is pain in the involved tissues. (If the tissues are rewarmed at this time, permanent injury can be avoided.) However, as the tissue freezes, all sensation is lost and the pain disappears.

Subsequently, the only symptom of frostbite may be the absence of any sensation in the frozen extremity. Such anesthesia may not be noticed by a victim who is involved in an activity such as climbing that claims all of his attention. The victim, aware only that the pain is gone, may think that his condition has improved, particularly if he is hypoxic from altitude or hypothermic and not thinking clearly.

However, the symptoms produced by frostbite are quite variable. Some individuals never experience pain; a few never lose it. A clear head and awareness of conditions that threaten frostbite are essential for its early recognition.

Frostbitten tissues are usually quite pale because the blood vessels are constricted and the amount of blood in the tissues is reduced. Frostbite of the nose or ears may be first noticed by someone other than the victim because the pallor can be seen. However, color changes in the hands or feet frequently go unnoticed because they are covered.

Frostbitten tissues also are usually firm or hard, although such changes may be limited to the superfical tissues. Sensation is typically absent in the involved tissues, particularly when the area is more than one inch (2.5 cm) in diameter.

If a large area, such as an entire foot or hand, is frostbitten, the tissues may appear purple as the result of sludging of blood within the vessels. That type of discoloration is an ominous finding that presages a loss of much or all of that portion of the extremity.

TREATMENT

The treatment for frostbite consists of rewarming the frozen tissues and minimizing the circulatory impairment that follows thawing.

Rewarming

The preferred treatment for frostbite is rapid rewarming in a water bath for which the temperature can be precisely controlled. Slow rewarming is associated with significantly greater tissue damage than rapid rewarming and should be avoided if possible. Rubbing the frostbitten tissues with snow or similar cold therapy was advocated during the Napoleonic campaigns because rapid rewarming by campfires or similar sources of dry heat had produced so much devastation. However, cold therapy aggravates the injury and must not be used. Dry heat from engine exhausts, open fires, or similar sources can not be controlled. Excessive temperatures are usually produced, resulting in a combined burn and frostbite, a devastating injury which leads to far greater tissue loss.

Rewarming of frostbitten feet should not be carried out in circumstances—such as a high altitude snow field—in which the victim must walk out under his own power. Once his feet have thawed, he will be unable to walk on them and will have to be carried.

No rewarming should be attempted until the victim has been evacuated to a situation in which there is no longer a significant possibility that the extremity might be refrozen. Thawing and refreezing does far more damage than walking on a frozen extremity.

Ideal situations for rapid rewarming are infrequently encountered. In urban surroundings frostbite victims are usually taken into a warm house until they can be transported to a hospital in a warm vehicle. By the time they reach the hospital the frostbitten tissues have thawed—slowly. The winter of 1976-1977 produced over 100 frostbite victims who sought medical assistance in Buffalo, New York. The typical delay before obtaining help was twelve to seventy-two hours.

In mountaineering situations the victim often must walk down below the snow line to reach a base camp or similar facility where rapid rewarming can be carried out. Frostbitten tissues often have thawed by the time he gets there.

Ideally, rewarming should not be carried out until the victim can be warmed to a normal body temperature and can be kept warm during rewarming and afterwards for as long as is required for recovery. When the body is cold, the blood vessels in the extremities are constricted. Rewarming frostbitten extremities in such circumstances would leave badly injured tissues without an adequate blood supply at the time it is most needed. Also, adequate facilities for prompt rewarming, including abundant supplies of warm water and methods for maintaining the temperature of the water bath, must be available. In less ideal situations prevention of slow thawing may be impossible. To limit tissue damage in such circumstances the frostbitten extremities should be rapidly rewarmed, even if optimal facilities are not available. However, if the toes or feet have been frozen, the climber will have to be carried to a point where motorized transportation is available.

For rewarming, any clothing or constricting items that could impair circulation, such as watch bands or rings, must be removed. The injured member should be suspended in the center of the bath and not permitted to rest against the side or bottom.

The water bath should be maintained at a temperature between 100° and 108° F (38° to 42° C). Hotter water would further damage the tissues. The water must not be hot enough to feel uncomfortable to an uninjured person's hand. A large water bath permits more accurate control of the temperature and may warm the frozen extremity more rapidly, probably resulting in less tissue loss.

A frostbitten hand or foot, like a block of ice, cools the water bath in which it is placed. The temperature of the bath must be maintained by adding warm water, not by heating the container. The victim's injured hand or foot could come in contact with the site to which heat was being applied and, because the tissues would be unable to feel the heat, a severe burn could result. The injured extremity should be removed from the bath when hot water is being added and should not be returned until the water has been thoroughly mixed and the temperature checked.

Warming usually requires twenty to forty minutes and should be continued until the tissues are soft and pliable. When rewarmed, frostbitten tissues that are destined to survive lose their pallor and take on a flushed appearance. Rewarming should be continued until no further improvement in color is being obtained.

Frostbitten tissues often become quite painful during rewarming. Aspirin or acetaminophen, alone or combined with codeine, or morphine, meperideine, or similar strong analgesics, may be administered to help control the pain. Some patients do not experience severe pain during rewarming, and for most the pain abates shortly afterwards.

Therapy to Improve Circulation

Since inadequacy of the blood supply to the frostbitten tissues appears to be responsible for much of the damage that results, efforts have been made to devise forms of therapy that would improve the circulation. Investigators who have found increased quantities of thromboxane and prostaglandins in the fluid of blisters that develop after rewarming have proposed treatment that would inhibit the release of these agents. This therapy still needs further controlled study to confirm its effectiveness, but the treatment is so simple, and significant side effects are so uncommon, that it seems to be worth trying in a wilderness situation. It consists simply of administering aspirin—common, ordinary aspirin. One or two tablets should be given while the tissues are still frozen and every six hours thereafter. (More of this drug would commonly be needed to help control pain.)

Other forms of treatment that have been tried are directed toward eliminating blood vessel constriction in the frostbitten tissues. The muscles in the walls of blood vessels are under the control of the autonomic, or involuntary, nervous system. The sympathetic nerves, one of the two major components of the autonomic nervous system, cause the muscles to contract and constrict the blood vessels. Parasympathetic nerves cause the muscles to relax and allow the vessels to dilate. Surgically cutting the sympathetic nerves to the frostbitten extremity has been found to modestly improve the outcome. However, such therapy is totally out of the question outside of a hospital.

Attempts have been made to achieve the same results pharmacologically by injecting the drug Reserpine, which blocks the sympathetic nerves, into the arteries supplying the frostbitten tissues. Results of this type of treatment have varied. Some physicians feel the treatment is beneficial; others have not found it helpful. Certainly the benefits are not outstanding. Moreover, intraarterial injections are difficult to perform, and individuals not experienced with such injections should not attempt them. Significant arterial injuries and severe bleeding can result. The drugs, syringes, and needles necessary for such injections would probably be carried only by a well equipped expedition or rescue group.

Additional Measures

After rewarming, the patient must be kept warm, and the injured tissues must be elevated and carefully protected from trauma or irritation. Sterile gauze or cotton should be placed between frostbitten fingers or toes to absorb moisture. Sleeping bags or bedclothes should be held off of frostbitten feet by some type of frame. Unless frostbitten tissues have been injured beyond recovery, large blisters develop on them after rewarming. Keeping the blisters intact reduces the risk of infection.

Usually the victim should be evacuated immediately. The only exceptions would be individuals with very minor injuries. Healing requires many weeks or months, depending upon the extent of the injury, and even more time is required to regain full use (if such is possible) of the extremity.

During evacuation, everything possible to prevent infection should be done. Cleanliness of the frostbitten area is vitally important. Soaking the extremity each day in disinfected, lukewarm water to which a germicidal soap has been added is helpful. Antibiotics probably should not be given routinely, but if infection appears to be present, and the patient is not allergic to penicillin, ampicillin or cloxicillin should be administered every six hours until a physician's care is obtained. Movement of the injured area, limited to that which can be performed voluntarily and without manipulation, should be encouraged. Cigarette smoking or other use of tobacco should be strictly prohibited because it further reduces the already deficient blood supply to the injured tissues.

Frostbite victims commonly suffer significant emotional reactions because they are faced with a long recovery and perhaps with severe permanent disability. Continuing reassurance and emotional support are a significant part of their nursing care.

Prognosis

The severity of frostbite injuries is notoriously difficult to judge accurately during the early stages. Such determinations may be almost impossible while the tissues are still frozen. Every physician who has cared for a significant number of frostbite victims has been surprised by individual patients whose final tissue loss has been greater or less than he expected. Sometimes, even the extent of the injury can not be determined accurately. However, purple discoloration of the tissue, instead of pallor, is commonly a sign of severe damage.

Following rewarming, several predictive signs appear. Rewarmed tissues develop a flushed appearance as the circulation is restored. Failure of the flush to appear or to extend to the tips of fingers or toes indicates that circulation has not been restored to those areas and that they probably will be lost. On areas of moderately severe frostbite blisters appear within a few hours to a few days after rewarming. Blisters filled with clear fluid that extend to the tips of the digits indicate the underlying tissues probably will recover. Blisters filled with bloody fluid, blisters that do not extend to the finger tips, or the failure of blisters to appear at all indicate that tissues are damaged beyond recovery. (Very minor frostbite injuries of the tips of digits, ears, or nose may not result in blisters after rewarming. The tissues may just turn red for a few days, although a crust may form and the superficial layer of skin may be lost.)

After a week or longer, dead frostbitten tissues develop a thick grey, dark green, or black covering called an eschar, which closely resembles the covering that develops over a third degree burn. In the ensuing weeks or months, fingers, toes, or other tissues which have been damaged beyond repair become black and mummified. Digits in such condition commonly separate or break off without surgery. Surgical intervention may be necessary if the tissues become infected (which is so common some physicians consider it almost unavoidable) or if a major portion of the hand or foot becomes mummified. Surgery also may be needed for reconstruction of the damaged extremities after they have separated.

ADDITIONAL READING

Fobson MC, Heggers JP: Evaluation of hand frostbite blister fluid as a clue to pathogenesis. *J Hand Surg* 1981;6:43-7.

McCauley RI, Hing DN, Robson MC, Heggers JP: Frostbite injuries: A rational approach based on the pathophysiology. *J Trauma* 1983;23:143-7.

Sumner DS, Criblez TL, and Doolittle WH: Host factors in human frostbite. *Milit Med* 1974;139:454-61.

CHAPTER EIGHT

Other Localized Cold Injuries

JAMES A. WILKERSON, M.D.

TRENCH FOOT

Trench foot is a type of localized cold injury which has occurred most commonly among foot soldiers during military operations. It apparently was first described during the Napoleonic campaigns but received its name during World War I from the men who spent weeks with their feet in the cold water that flooded the trenches. During that conflict, the British had over 115,000 casualties due to trench foot and frostbite. During the Second World War, the Americans had approximately 60,000 trench foot casualties, eighty-five percent of them among infantry rifle companies. Only fifteen percent of the casualties eventually returned to combat. During the worst part of the harsh 1944-1945 winter, particularly during the German counteroffensive known as "The Battle of the Bulge," trench foot accounted for one-third of the battlefield casualties admitted to general hospitals in the Paris area. Identical injuries among victims of sea warfare who spent days with their feet in the cold water of cramped, partially flooded lifeboats and liferafts, led to the name "immersion foot."

Trench foot remains a devastating injury for soldiers in cold, wet weather. In the Falkland Islands fighting, seventy of the 516 British battle casualties requiring hospitalization were victims of trench foot. Estimates of the number who had significant injuries but did not require hospitalization ranged as high as 2,000. None of the British casualties required amputation, an indication of the early and excellent care they received on the hospital ships. Reportedly, the Argentinian forces, who did not have such medical facilities available, had a far larger number of trench foot injuries and many amputations.

96

Footsoldiers of both forces were forced to lie for days in flooded trenches or were repeatedly soaked by freezing rain and chilled by forty to sixty knot winds, which are nearly hurricane force (46 to 69 mph or 74 to 111 kph).

"Trench foot" is probably the most widely known name for this disorder. "Immersion foot" is sometimes considered more appropriate, but several different immersion syndromes have been recognized, and the similarity of their names tends to be confusing. Since trench foot, like frostbite, is a localized cold injury, but the tissues are not frozen, "nonfreezing localized cold injury" is undoubtedly the most appropriate name for this disorder but is too cumbersome for common use.

Mechanism of Injury

Trench foot is produced by many days or even weeks of continuously wet feet in near freezing weather. Actual immersion of the feet in water is not necessary; continuously wet socks and boots in association with cold weather can be just as damaging. In such situations two mechanisms greatly reduce the temperature of the tissues of the feet. First, the circulation of blood to the lower extremities is reduced because the victim's body is cold and the peripheral blood vessels have constricted to reduce heat loss. Second, the cold water with which the feet are in contact extracts much of the remaining heat from the tissues and causes further vasoconstriction. The result is an extremely cold extremity with a greatly reduced blood supply.

Prolonged cooling damages the tissues. The marked reduction in blood circulation probably contributes, but does not appear to directly cause injury to the tissues as occurs with frostbite. The injury that results is not the same as that caused by obstruction of the blood supply.

All of the tissues are damaged, but the most common crippling injuries are those to nerves. Nerve damage is responsible for the pain, the prickling or tingling sensations (paresthesias), or the total anesthesia which may result. Damage to the skin is evidenced by a red color, the development of blisters—which may be large (blebs)—and by bleeding into the skin (ecchymoses). Damage to the other tissues is indicated by swelling.

Prevention

Trench foot can be prevented by avoiding wet feet for prolonged periods of time in a cold environment. During the First World War, the British dropped their rate of cold injury from 33.9 cases per thousand men in 1914 to 3.8 cases per thousand in 1918 by implementing three simple rules: first, every soldier was required to have a spare pair of socks; second, arrangements for drying and reissue of socks during tours in the trenches were mandatory; and third, boots and socks had to be removed, the feet dried and massaged well (to promote circulation), and dry socks put on as circumstances allowed. Officers were charged with the responsibility for enforcing the preventive measures in their units.

During active combat, avoiding being killed is undoubtedly more pressing than caring for wet feet. In some battlefield situations drying the feet or any part of the body may be impossible. However, awareness of the potential for disabling injury from prolonged exposure to wet and cold should lead officers and the men for whom they are responsible to take preventive measures whenever an opportunity can be found. Simply putting on dry socks and drying the boots as well as possible will help avoid trench foot or at least greatly reduce its severity.

Outdoorsmen who are not in combat would rarely if ever have their feet wet and cold for days at a time. Fishermen, waterfowl hunters, white water enthusiasts, and high altitude climbers using vapor impermeable boots appear to be at greatest risk for such injuries, but even if their feet were wet throughout the day they could be dried and warmed at night. Simple awareness of the potential for injury by prolonged cold water immersion should prompt adequate protective measures.

Diagnosis

The earliest symptoms of trench foot among the British soldiers in the Falklands were variable. For some the first evidence of this disorder was numbness, which generally appeared after seven to ten days. Others had paresthesias (prickling or tingling sensations, or feelings like electric shocks) which made sleep difficult. For some, pain was the initial symptom and also caused problems with sleep. Pain which was almost unbearable upon first putting weight on the feet in the morning was typical. The symptoms tended to spread slowly upwards.

The earliest visible sign of injury is redness of the skin. With greater damage the tissues become swollen (edematous). In the Falklands, feet were commonly so swollen that soldiers had difficulty putting on their boots in the morning. With more severe injuries the feet become quite red, greater swelling is present, and large blisters develop. Such changes are usually associated with severe sensory abnormalities. Rarely, the feet become obviously dead or gangrenous.

A combination of two classifications of the severity of trench foot developed during World War II is listed in Table 7.

Table 7. Features of Trench Foot of Different Severities

Grade	Characteristic Features
Minimal	Reddening of the skin; slight sensory change
Mild	Swelling; sensory changes (reversible)
Moderate	Swelling, redness, blebs, and intracutaneous hemorrhage; irreversible nerve damage
Severe	Severe swelling, blebs, massive bleeding into the skin and other tissues; gangrene

Treatment

Little treatment of trench foot is possible; usually little is necessary. The most widely used measures consist of keeping the feet clean and dry and keeping them elevated to help relieve the swelling. The patient must be kept warm so the feet can have a generous blood supply .

For more severe injuries, debridement, resection of portions of the foot, or even amputation may be necessary, but such treatment must be carried out by experienced surgeons in a hospital setting.

Prognosis

Most patients recover completely from trench foot, although many have a permanent reduced tolerance for cold. Most of the British soldiers in the Falklands had completely recovered by the time their troopships had returned to Great Britain, or by three and one-half months after the end of the fighting. However, studies of randomly selected soldiers found that many did have damaged nerves (de-myelinated medial or lateral plantar nerves). Also, many had residual cold sensitivity evidenced by marked vascular constriction in response to only moderate cold stimuli, and a tendency for the constriction to persist in spite of rewarming. Whether troops injured by cold can be effective again in a cold environment remains to be answered.

Individuals who require surgery would be disabled if an extensive resection or amputation is necessary. A few individuals have required amputation for intractable pain caused by nerve damage months or years after the initial injury.

OTHER TYPES OF IMMERSION INJURY

Warm Water Immersion Foot

Soldiers in Viet Nam and other campaigns have developed injuries from prolonged, intermittent immersion of their feet in warm water. The wrinkling of the soles of the feet typical of water immersion for a few minutes is greatly exaggerated if the feet are exposed to intermittent wetness for three to ten days. As a result, the soles of the feet become swollen and painful, particularly over the weight bearing areas on the heels and balls of the foot.

If the victim is put to bed with his feet exposed to air so they stay dry, most of the visible changes will disappear within twenty-four hours. Most of the symptoms will clear within two weeks.

This type of injury is not a cold injury, as is trench foot. Warm water immersion injury is probably produced by trauma to the skin on the sole of a foot that already has been softened, and perhaps damaged, by prolonged wetness.

Paddy Foot

Another type of warm water immersion injury affects the skin of the tops of the feet and the lower legs. This injury results from almost continuous—rather than intermittent—wetness of the feet for forty-eight to sixty hours. The first symptom is itching, which is followed by the appearance of numerous small blisters, redness, bleeding into the skin, a dull aching with walking, and swelling of the foot which leaves it hard (nonpitting edema). Most of the victims can not walk. According to one report, twenty percent of the soldiers constantly in water for seventy-two hours, and eighty percent of those constantly in water for 120 hours, were incapacitated.

Drying the feet and keeping them elevated is the only treatment needed. Most victims have been able to return to duty in forty-eight hours.

Although this disorder results from prolonged immersion, it also is not a cold injury.

CHILBLAINS

Chilblains is a nonfreezing cold injury which is uncomfortable, but causes little or no impairment. This disorder results from repeated exposure of bare skin to wet, windy conditions at temperatures ranging from 60° F (15.5° C) to near freezing. It commonly occurs on the hands, cheeks, or knees of persons inadequately clothed for such weather. Acute chilblains is characterized by red, warm, tender, swollen, and itchy (pruritic) skin. In the more common chronic stage the skin is red, rough, and cool to the touch. Drying and cracking are typical.

Treatment consists of the application of a bland, moisterizing ointment to the injured skin. Warm, protective clothing should be worn to prevent recurrences or worsening of the condition.

ADDITIONAL READING

Akers WA: Paddy foot: A warm water immersion foot syndrome variant. *Mili Med* 1974; 139:605-618.

Marsh AR: A short but distant war—the Falklands Campaign. *J Roy Soc Med* 1983; 76:972-982.

APPENDIX

Thermometers that can measure body temperatures as low as 75° to 80°F (24° to 27° C) are produced by the following companies:

Carolina Biological Products
P.O. Box 187
Gladstone, Oregon 97027

Dynamed, Inc.
6200 Yarrow Drive
Carlsbad, California 92008

Zeal G.H., Ltd.
8 Lombard Street
London, S.W. 19, England

Index

NOTES

NOTES

NOTES

NOTES

NOTES

NOTES

NOTES

NOTES

Other books from The Mountaineers include:

The ABC of AVALANCHE SAFETY, Second Edition, by Ed LaChapelle. Classic pocket-sized handbook on avalanche basics and rescue; for all types of snow-country travelers.

MEDICINE FOR MOUNTAINEERING, Fourth Edition, James A. Wilkerson, MD, editor. A handbook of medicine, compiled by climber-physicians, for treatment of traumatic, environmental and high-altitude injuries, illnesses, in remote areas.

MOUNTAINEEERING FIRST AID, Third Edition, by Marty Lentz, Jan Carline, Steven Macdonald. Basics of immediate care, prevention of outdoor accidents and illnesses. Follows format of mountaineering-oriented first aid classes.

MOUNTAINEERING: The Freedom of the Hills, Fifth Edition, Don Graydon, editor. Most complete, up-to-date book in existence on how to climb. Standard text for all mountaineering classes.

Write for illustrated catalog of more than 300 outdoor titles:

The Mountaineers • Books
1011 S.W. Klickitat Way, Seattle, WA 98134
(800) 553-4453